BIRTHING ROOMS

Concept and reality

Y0-BDW-855

SOUTHERN MISSIONARY COLLEGE
Division of Nursing Library
711 Lake Estelle Drive
Orlando, Florida 32803

DF 9013
nursing
anesthesia

BIRTHING ROOMS
Concept and reality

PHILIP E. SUMNER, M.D., F.A.C.O.G.

Manchester Memorial Hospital,
Manchester, Connecticut

CELESTE R. PHILLIPS, R.N., M.S.

Instructor, Mission College,
Santa Clara, California

Editorial consultants

Samuel Smith, M.D.
John Wheeler, M.D.

with 80 illustrations

WQ
27.1
.S956
1981

9630

The C. V. Mosby Company

ST. LOUIS • TORONTO • LONDON   1981

SOUTHERN MISSIONARY COLLEGE
Division of Nursing Library
711 Lake Estelle Drive
Orlando, Florida 32803

MOSBY

1906 **75** 1981
YEARS

A TRADITION OF PUBLISHING EXCELLENCE

Copyright © 1981 by The C. V. Mosby Company

All rights reserved. No part of this book may be reproduced
in any manner without written permission of the publisher.

Printed in the United States of America

The C. V. Mosby Company
11830 Westline Industrial Drive, St. Louis, Missouri 63141

Library of Congress Cataloging in Publication Data

Sumner, Philip E., 1925-
    Birthing rooms, concept and reality.

    Bibliography: p.
    Includes index.
    1.   Hospitals, Gynecologic and obstetric.   2.   Child-
birth.   3.   Manchester Memorial Hospital.   I.   Phillips,
Celeste R., 1933-   II.   Title.   [DNLM: 1.   Hospital
departments.   2.   Obstetrics.   3.   Natural childbirth.
WQ 27.1 S956b]
RG500.S95   362.1′982   81-993
ISBN 0-8016-4873-4   AACR2

C/D/D   9   8   7   6   5   4   3   2   1   02/C/225

To
our families
Roger, Duncan, and **Catherine Phillips**
Margi, Smokey, and **Jeff Sumner**

Foreword

Today, many people think that the family is doomed. In spite of the prognosis of doom an entirely new approach to childbirth has occurred within the last 20 years. It is the idea of participatory childbirth, of a family-directed childbirth, which seems to have not only influenced but also practically revolutionized obstetric attitudes and thinking as well as hospital procedures. There was no smooth transition from thinking of anesthetizing the woman as the norm and best way to handle childbirth to accepting, supporting, and finally encouraging an awake, aware, and participating woman in childbirth. It has been a thorny road for adherents to this new idea. As recently as 5 to 8 years ago prepared childbirth was considered a fad that was bound to be short lived and would quietly disappear. But contrary to so many people's expectations, the concept of being a conscious participant in the birth of one's child not only became a way of life with those who were fighting for it but also was accepted by the medical and nursing professions as a sound and viable alternative to childbirth with drugs. This idea has been incorporated into our literature and the performing arts, in films and on the stage.

The movement toward a shared childbirth experience started as a consumer movement, and it has continued as such until the present. It is the parents, the families who proselytize and demand healthy and joyful birthing experiences, with the help of a team of health care providers: the physician, the nurse, the childbirth educator, and often the monitrice.

Families and parents do not, however, act and live in a vacuum. The general climate in the Western world and the thinking of the 1960s generation have been toward a simpler life, ecology, rediscovery of basic and natural resources, and a movement away from impersonal technology. In the last 20 years ideas have been directed toward redefining human values and human experiences.

It was no coincidence that three of the most influential organizations in the field of childbirth education were formed 20 years ago. They are the ASPO (American Society for Psychoprophylaxis in Obstetrics, Inc.), ICEA (International Childbirth Education Association), and La Leche League. All three are representatives and spokespeople for the family in our time.

During the same 20 years giant steps were made in the obstetric field. Obstetrics became a science, where electronic devices brought great advances to medicine and made the event of childbirth safer than it had ever been for both mother and baby. However, the introduction of intricate technology and the advances in medical knowledge caused pregnancy and childbirth to be regarded as an illness of which a woman had to be cured. It was not that the professionals disliked treating each woman according to her own needs; in fact, their medical training urges them to do just that. But it is difficult to combine sophisticated technology with human warmth and empathy, particularly in surroundings that are geared to treat pathologic conditions, surroundings that are built for efficiency, for safe and sterile procedures. At present the vast majority of women are expected to give birth in such environments.

It is therefore very reassuring to know that dialogues between the educated consumer and the professional team have begun to take place—the professional, interested in safety and efficiency, the consumer, in human values. One concept and approach does not necessarily exclude the other. It is because of this dialogue that Dr. Philip Sumner, scientist and obstetrician, Celeste R. Phillips, nurse and educator, and the parents who were active participants came together to write this important book, which shows the way for science and humanity to become partners.

I have known Dr. Sumner for many years. He is a humanist who had the courage of his conviction. He introduced the concept of the birthing room, with its comfortable, pleasant, and safe surroundings, not just for a few privileged women but for every family. Through his ideas and work Dr. Sumner became a part of the team that allows for safety in childbirth, which none of us wants to give up, and at the same time safeguards the feelings, joys, and close ties of modern families.

I do not think that the new approach to childbirth or the twentieth century family is in danger of disappearing, not as long as physicians, nurses, childbirth educators, and parents are equal partners in the fight for safety and preservation of human values.

By sharing his 11 years of experience, Dr. Sumner shows that a modern maternity can function in any setting, be it a community hospital, a large university, or a large city clinic.

Elisabeth Bing

Preface

As this book is being written, there is growing consumer protest over increasingly more active management of childbirth with new technology. Conferences are being held throughout the United States to discuss alternatives to technologic birth. More and more couples are boycotting the existing medical system and are choosing to give birth at home. Many providers of health care are responding to consumer pressure by offering alternatives to home birth within the hospital system, usually with highly structured and well-defined risk criteria that tend to make them available only to a select population.

We believe that such measures, although commendable and long overdue, are only part of the answer. At the core of the problem is consumer dissatisfaction with the attitudes of those attending families during pregnancy, labor, and birth. Acceptance of birth as a normal physiologic process for all families can begin by institutions demystifying and simplifying the birth ritual.

This book is about a hospital setting in which childbirth for all families is a normal and creative event. The program at this hospital has a number of distinctive features: (1) physical and emotional preparation of the mother and father, (2) a single, all-inclusive unit for both labor and birth, with all mothers eligible for this unit, (3) availability of continuous, one-to-one support for mother and father throughout labor and delivery by a maternity nurse (monitrice) prepared in psychoprophylaxis, and (4) individualization of each birth experience with maximum emotional support for the new family.

Forming a philosophic basis for this program are the following premises with regard to childbirth and its management.

1. The sensitivity and humanity of a society are reflected in its childbirth practices.
2. Western society urgently needs to define certain basic humane, philosophic guidelines for childbirth.
3. The definition of childbirth is critical, since how we define childbirth will determine how we treat it.

     a. Pregnancy defined and managed as an illness and birth as an operation (vaginal or abdominal) create a negative orientation: morbidity, pathology, passivity, austerity, and sterility.

     b. Pregnancy defined and managed as a normal physiologic process and birth as a normal physiologic event and a peak emotional experience create a positive orientation: healthiness, activity, work, joy, beauty, love, and fulfillment.

4. There is no one right way to manage childbirth. Many different models have equal validity; however, the essential elements must include medical safety and emotional fulfillment. Birth represents the creation of a new human spirit, and therefore the opportunity for some form of spiritual expression is important.

5. The family is the basic unit of our society. Each family member is entitled to recognition and consideration. Childbearing is an important function of the family to be shared together.

6. The mother's own mechanism of labor, cultivated and strengthened by education and training through a prepared childbirth program, should be the cornerstone of modern obstetric management.

7. Each labor is unique and requires individualized management. *Routine* procedures such as perineal preparation, enema, intravenous therapy, electronic fetal monitoring, medication, anesthesia, forceps usage, episiotomy, and manual removal of placenta may represent excessive obstetric *intervention*.

8. Labor-delivery–postpartum period is a single, continuous event and is appropriately managed in a single location, such as a birthing room.

9. Uninterrupted, one-to-one support of the childbearing family by an experienced and knowledgeable obstetric nurse (monitrice) helps to minimize the need for drugs and maximize the positive experience of birth.

10. Since the majority of women have normal, uncomplicated pregnancies and births, the local community hospital can meet most families' birthing needs.

11. The hospital can serve as an educational center for professional and lay childbirth and parenting groups.

12. Because emergencies requiring immediate and skilled medical and nursing management can suddenly arise, hospital births are safer than out-of-hospital births.

13. Cultivation of responsible parenting in the immediate postpartum period is an important part of the birth experience.

14. It is important that all members of an obstetric team share the same basic philosophy about the management of childbirth. However, there is *no one right way* to have a baby, and since the practice of obstetrics is both an *art* and a *science*, each situation must be individualized according to the needs of the family and the mother's obstetric situation.

We hope that this book will contribute to the achievement of a blending of both our technologic and humanitarian advances to benefit yet unborn genera-tions.

Philip Sumner
Celeste Phillips

Notes to the reader

In 1969, Manchester Memorial Hospital became the first hospital in the United States to establish a birth room. Manchester, located in central Connecticut, has a population of about 50,000 composed mainly of Irish and Italian ethnic groups. Less than 3% of the population are black or Hispanic. Many of the people in the community are employed in Hartford, a large city 6 miles to the west. Although the industrial area in Manchester is enlarging, it is not a primarily industrial town.

Manchester Memorial Hospital is a 300-bed community hospital located in central Manchester. It has 24 maternity beds with 12 pediatricians and ten obstetricians on the staff, all utilizing the hospital birth rooms.

I will admit that in my first few hours at Manchester Memorial Hospital, I was disappointed with what I saw. I had traveled to Connecticut expecting to find a hospital alternative birth center like those in northern California where I live. However, I did not find hospital rooms decorated just like home, with double beds for mom and dad. Instead, I saw small, comfortable-looking birthing rooms with a labor-delivery bed, a bright light source, and low-profile medical equipment, such as a Kreisselman crib.

I had visited enough hospital alternative birth centers by this time to realize that no two were alike. The decor of the room is limited only by the amount of money the hospital is able to spend. And, just as decor varies in hospital birth centers, policies, procedures, and protocols vary. However, one common thread ran through all the hospital birth centers I had visited: only very low-risk women were admitted to them. In fact, most of the hospitals used the term "alternative" birth rooms, meaning a hospital system's alternative to home birth. Unfortunately, I have often felt that the primary motivation for the establishment of many hospital birthing rooms is financial, perhaps to recover money lost through families choosing to give birth at home, or in birth centers outside of hospitals. In these centers the controlling attitude of staff had not changed and the birth room differed in name only. In reality, the staff clung to rigid routine procedures and thought of birth as pathologic, quickly emphasizing the "risks" couples took by choosing alternative birth centers.

So what was different about Manchester Memorial and Philip Sumner? My first clue was that the birthing room concept had been a reality there since 1969, approximately 5 years before the alternative birth movement began. Childbirth there had been recognized and supported as a physiologic event and peak emotional experience long before doing so was fashionable. But my biggest surprise came when I asked Dr. Sumner what his screening criteria were for use of the birth rooms. He answered that *all* women could give birth in the birth rooms, except those needing cesarean birth or difficult obstetric procedures. There were no risk criteria. What had started cautiously in 1969 as one birthing room (Lamaze room) limited to women trained in the psychoprophylactic method with a monitrice had evolved into a way for all women to give birth, prepared or unprepared, high risk or healthy. This was *not* an alternative to home birth, but a joyous model for giving birth in a hospital setting. It worked. Philip Sumner and his colleagues had proven that in over 10 years and over 4000 births.

Celeste Phillips

Manchester Memorial Hospital is now planning to build a totally new, family-centered maternity unit. As part of predevelopment planning, Dr. Sumner composed the following statement regarding the childbirth philosophy and policies of the new unit:

Throughout the country maternity units of general hospitals are coming under increasing consumer pressure to develop childbirth policies and procedures which will humanize and dignify the birthing process and enable the young parents to take an active and meaningful part in this important family experience. The concept of family-centered maternity care has been developed to meet this need by modifying traditional attitudes and policies, and encouraging each member of the nuclear family to participate and share in all phases of the birthing process.

Since 1969 when it opened the first birthing room in the country, Manchester Memorial Hospital has been committed to and actively engaged in the development of a flexible, humanized, family-oriented childbirth program. The goal of this program is to offer expectant couples that method of childbirth which best meets their individual needs and aspirations. What began as a small "clinical experiment" at Manchester Memorial Hospital, with the establishment of a single birthing room in which an occasional "prepared" couple could both labor and deliver, has now grown to a major obstetric movement in which the majority of women give birth using one of our three "birthing rooms." In 1978, over 700 of the approximately 1300 births at our hospital took place in the birthing rooms. Manchester Memorial Hospital's birthing program recognizes the importance of individualized and humanized childbirth at reasonable cost, while at the same time providing the full resources of medical technology. This birthing center recognizes the fact that, for most women, childbirth is fundamentally a normal, uncomplicated physiological event, and not a disease process. This center recognizes and manages childbirth as a joyous, creative, human, family event, and not as a pathologic, high-risk medical or surgical event like pneumonia or appendicitis.

Prior to the late 1960s, childbirth was often managed in a routine "assembly line" manner, with women unprepared, frightened, and passive, and fathers excluded. Mothers were transferred from the early labor room, to the advanced labor room, to the delivery room, to the recovery room, to the postpartum room. Medication and anesthesia, intravenous therapy, Pitocin stimulation, forceps, etc., were routinely used and the baby was "delivered" by the obstetrician. Today with the rapid growth of the prepared childbirth movement and the increasing demands of the consumer to make the experience of childbirth not only safe, but also emotionally meaningful and rewarding, traditional childbirth philosophies and policies are becoming obsolete. The birthing center concept offers an appropriate facility to more fully meet the different needs of the awake, aware, and actively participating mothers who "give birth." It offers conventional labor and delivery facilities for those who choose to have their deliveries in the traditional manner, or whose attendants may prefer the regular delivery room. It also offers the usual operating rooms in the event that a cesarean delivery must be performed. However, the emphasis of the program is on labor-delivery rooms (birth rooms) and the availability of optional, one-to-one nursing support (monitrice) throughout labor and delivery. Postpartum facilities are oriented to strengthening the family unit through nonseparation and active participation in all phases of baby care. The birthing center is primarily oriented to healthy pregnant mothers who constitute the vast majority of pregnant women, but who have been neglected in the past by the obstetric community in favor of the small minority of pregnant women who are having complicated pregnancies. However, since modern medical technology is available, the birthing center is also appropriate to manage the intermediate-risk mother, who may be having more difficult labor, and even many of the women classified as high risk. Although Manchester Memorial Hospital does not have its own intensive care unit for newborns, it is able to offer a full range of simple and sophisticated obstetric services for both mother and child through the coordinated consortium program of immediate consultation and transfer when necessary. Birthing rooms are available for all laboring women, whether they have attended prepared childbirth classes or not. The Manchester Memorial Family Birthing Center is not a hospital program alone, but rather a combined community program. The hospital acts as a central coordinator while professional and lay organizations work together to offer a thorough and comprehensive program of prenatal, natal, and postnatal services of far greater scope than could be offered by the hospital or medical and nursing professions alone. Family-centered childbirth requires a *team* approach, which includes the mother and father, other family members, the obstetrician, pediatrician, family physician, certified nurse-midwife, monitrice, hospital staff nurses, nurse practitioners, childbirth educators, and other health providers. It is our conviction that this coordinated team effort enables the expectant couple to become better educated, prepared, and motivated for childbirth and responsible parenthood. Such preparation enables them to have a safe and satisfying childbirth experience, tailored to meet their individual needs in a humanized hospital environment. Through this combined community effort, the Manchester Memorial Family Birthing Center offers various aspects of family-centered care, which include: (1) prenatal education, (2) nutritional consultation, (3) physical and emotional preparation for birth and parenting, (4) elimination of routines and risk criteria for eligibility, (5) individualization of patient management, (6) father participation in labor, birth, and baby care, (7) helpful interaction on an individualized basis to facilitate labor and delivery, (8) emphasis on noninvasive, multiple support techniques, instead of primary reliance on intervention techniques such as drugs, anesthetics, IVs, and forceps, (9) the importance of humanized, one-to-one support by an experienced obstetric nurse (monitrice) throughout labor, delivery, and the first hour post partum, (10) nontransfer of the mother for delivery, (11) sensitivity, beauty, and dignity of the birth scene (dimming of lights, gentle handling, bathing, skin-to-skin contact, eye-to-eye contact, breastfeeding, withholding of silver nitrate and other drugs), (12) recognition of the importance of the complex, meaningful interaction of the new nuclear family in the birthing room, and later during the postpartum period, with attention to rooming-in, sibling visitation, and intense education of both parents in infant care, and (13) all the other important nurturing activities on the part of a sensitive and caring hospital nursing staff.

We believe the Manchester experience may suggest to other hospital obstetric services in the United States a possible model for individualizing and dignifying childbirth without compromising safety. It is a basic, flexible model that is applicable for both prepared childbirth families and those who have not prepared for birth. This model can easily be modified to adapt to the individual circumstances of each hospital's unique situation. Although clearly there can be no one best model, and many different models may have equal validity, it is nevertheless our sincere belief that this is one clinically-proven program that embodies certain universal principles of childbirth. These basics have the potential to change obstetric management from a *pathologic* orientation to a *humanistic* experience that can strengthen positive parenting.

Although we realize that achieving the optimum in maternity care will require continual research and review, we offer the Manchester experience as one model that strives to achieve a safe and humanized in-hospital childbirth experience for all.

Acknowledgments

A book such as this would never have happened without the work of the giants in the field of prepared childbirth: doctors such as Dick-Read, Velvovsky, Lamaze, Vellay, Chabon, and Bradley; teachers and leaders such as Elisabeth Bing, Marjorie Karmel, Sheila Kitzinger, Ferris Urbanowski, Flora Hommel, and Melba Gandy; and the American Society for Psychoprophylaxis in Obstetrics board of directors. Their fine work was inspirational.

To translate that inspiration into clinical reality required a great deal of blood, sweat, and tears. The fine people who contributed so much to the latter include: my two partners, Dr. John Wheeler and Dr. Samuel Smith, whose 100% enthusiastic support of our program has enabled us to speak with one voice; our two great nurse practitioners, Billy Carlson and Irma Meridy; and our dedicated office staff members Arlene Stryjeski, Alice Belcher, Genie Arvisais, Kathy Bittner, Sandy Smith, and Joanne Pitz, who keep peace in our office where otherwise pandemonium would prevail.

Each member of the Manchester Monitrice Associates has contributed greatly to our program, but Sandy Eckstrom, Billy Carlson, Marcia Memery, Marilyn Hull, Sue Moore, Kathy Chmielecki, Ida Anderson, and Barbara Soderberg have been involved from the beginning. To them we owe so much, for without them our program could not exist.

I should especially like to acknowledge the unswerving support and fair-mindedness of our hospital administrator, Edward Kenney, who from the beginning allowed all philosophies of childbirth to have equal expression. Thanks are also due to Robert Smith and his hard-working board of trustees for their constant support and encouragement. Also, I would like to express my deep appreciation to the John DeQuattro family for their generous contributions, which enabled us to properly equip our birthing rooms. The ongoing support and cooperation from Frances Surowiec, Head Nurse, and Carol Hunt, Nursing Supervisor, and the loyal, dedicated staff nurses at Manchester Memorial Hospital have been essential to the "team effort" and the success of the program. Sincere appreciation is extended to all of these fine nurses as well as to my obstetric colleagues who, although not always agreeing with what we were doing, granted us the right to do it.

As to the actual writing of this book, I am most thankful to Riekie Ehrlich, who years ago gave me the initial encouragement to undertake this task; to Margi, my wife, who has not only had to put up with the usual erratic hours of a busy obstetrician, but also has given up the few hours we would normally share so that I could devote time to this book; and last but not least to my hard-working coauthor, Celeste Phillips, who has devoted endless hours of creative talent and effort to strengthening and expanding this book from a simple narrative of a clinical program to a broad examination and presentation of progressive childbirth concepts, which we hope will make at least a small contribution to all of those disciplines concerned with the improvement of the experience of birth.

Philip Sumner

We also acknowledge the contributions to this book made by friends and fellow travelers on the road to humanizing birth. Sandra Aylsworth contributed Chapter 1 on the History of birth environments; we appreciate her historical perspective. Marcia Memery spent long hours interviewing couples and then typing pages of material for Chapter 3. In addition to this excellent contribution, Marcia and her husband, Jim Memery, are responsible for taking and developing photographs of those couples interviewed, the monitrice group, Drs. Wheeler and Smith, and the paracervical block setup. Eileen Comeau did a beautiful job in compiling the data from 2830 births recorded in the Lamaze Log and then typing a synthesis of the Manchester program.

In the final chapter, experiences in developing alternatives to traditional birth were contributed by nurses Vicky Peterson, Carolyn Fisher, Renetta Parris, and Ruth Watson Lubic, and Drs. Anthony Damore, Joseph Anzalone, and Joseph D'Amico. Ruth Watson Lubic, in her role of General Director and Assistant Secretary to the Maternity Center Association in New York, was especially helpful.

For typing the manuscript we are very appreciative of the work of Catherine Nagel and Elsie Ciapponi. However, all the inspiration and work of those professionals acknowledged here would mean nothing without the parents—the families who granted us the right to translate inspiration into reality. To the families whose remarkable and beautiful experiences have been the catalyst for this book, we are forever grateful. These are the people who have made it all possible.

And last, but certainly not least, we want to thank Nancy Evans, former Senior Editor of Nursing Science at The C. V. Mosby Co. Because she recognized that we shared a common dream, we met across a continent, and this book became a reality.

Celeste Phillips
Philip Sumner

Contents

CHAPTER 1

Birth environments: historical background

Sandra Aylsworth, M.A. in History

Although the physical process of birth has been the same as long as human beings have existed, the settings for this experience have varied widely. Just as the alternative birth movement today reflects modern conditions, a study of birth environments throughout time reflects changes in society. A complete understanding of the Manchester experience and other birthing trends is aided by studying the places of birth over the centuries.

PRIMITIVE SOCIETIES

The stereotype of birth in primitive societies is of the female giving birth wherever she was at the time; she simply squatted during the second stage of labor, cut the umbilical cord with her teeth, and resumed work after the expulsion of the placenta. Some sociologists, however, have suggested that just as a cat finds a warm, dry place to be alone, the earliest women withdrew to a secluded part of the cave or forest when their time came. Instinct was their only assistant.

Women probably began attending each other during birth as early as the Paleolithic or Early Stone Age in environments close to their homes. Groups were small, and so the few adult women could not be spared from their regular tasks for long. Any great distance from the group would have necessitated more effort to provide shelter from the elements and protection from wild animals. The choices were therefore limited.

As agriculture developed and settled communities were established, local taboos and rituals influenced the selection of a birth environment and attendants. The idea of parturients being unclean predates the famous Old Testament rites of purification. The fear of blood found in many cultures was one reason women had to remove themselves from the group for birth. Sometimes special structures were built by the community, the father, or the women.

In preliterate Siam (now called Thailand), birth took place in a special room to which the mother of a firstborn was confined for 30 days. She had to expose her naked abdomen and back to a constantly burning fire as part of a sacrificial purification.

Huron and Iroquois mothers were not supposed to give birth in their own houses; they were secluded for 40 days in a small structure outside the village. Birth beside a stream was often favored so that the mother could wash herself and the baby. Other groups dug holes into the floor of the structure where loose earth could receive discharges. Aromatic herbs were sometimes present to make the atmosphere more pleasant and for magical purposes.

Men and fathers

Men have been excluded from the childbirth environment in many cultures; some hospitals still discourage the presence of the father in the delivery room. The Ik people of the mountains of Uganda prohibit the father from even entering his own house until a week after the birth, when the baby is publicly displayed.

In the Trobriand Islands of the southwest Pacific, as late as the 1940s no men were allowed to enter the house where a mother and her newborn were confined for the first month. A small fire was kept burning under the raised bedstead as a prophylactic against black magic. Bronislaw Malinowski's 1922 anthropologic classic explained that they had no word for father and did not recognize the connection between intercourse and conception. In this matrilineal society the father established his role by sharing in the care of the children, cleaning the baby, and holding him in his arms to feed him mashed vegetables.

The women of the Herero, a Bantu-speaking group of southwestern Africa, build a special hut for the parturient, whom men are not allowed to see until the navel string has separated from the infant. The men believe that seeing her before this time will make them weaklings.

Other primitive groups allowed men to be present at the birth process. In *Eternal Eve* Harvey Graham[2] describes natives of the Brazilian interior. An Indian woman of the Caraya tribe would squat and grab an outdoor post or tree; her husband would squat behind her and use his hands to press on the contracting womb. He would tie and bite the umbilical cord. In other Brazilian tribes the father would paint the infant with red and black pigments before placing him in a special bed.

In the Sandwich Islands (now called Hawaii), one method was for the parturient to sit on the lap of an old man (not her own husband) and deliver in public. Husbands were usually present at births in the Lapland and American Indian cultures, but an older woman with experience was the most involved birth attendant.

Husbands were more likely to participate when difficulties arose. In one area of old Hungary, the husband would assist only if labor was prolonged. He would shake his wife three times and have her drink three times out of his left palm. She would then kick the floor three times with her left heel. The husband would help the midwife bathe the laboring woman and tie his own waistband around her body three times. He was dismissed immediately after the birth. In Serbia (now part of Yugoslavia), a drink of water from the husband's boot was considered helpful.

Birth environments

Just as today, the welfare of the mother and child influenced the selection of a birth environment in primitive societies. Demons were to be avoided, propitiated or frightened away. This sometimes meant noise and a lack of privacy. In east Africa, drummers might accompany the parturient to ward off evil spirits. After giving birth, women in some cultures rushed out of the birth hut and flailed the air with weapons. Elsewhere, a slow procession around the lying-in structure included the mother carrying her child while a great commotion was made with bells and palm branches. Fires, even though not needed for heat, have often been part of the birth scene, perhaps a carry-over from ancient times when roaming carnivores were a threat. Some cultures still keep a candle burning in the birthing room.

The Pygmies of the Congo had a casual, almost carefree attitude toward childbirth. Other children were allowed to enter the birth hut if they wished. The man could be present at the birth but could not sleep with a nursing mother.

A Chinese birth environment traditionally included a low bed on which the parturient sat with her back against a wall, and a brick under each foot. One task of the attending midwife was to keep "four-eyed persons" (a term used for pregnant women) away. The new mother and her baby had to remain in that same house for a month because the postpartum discharge was considered a polluting substance. All birth fluids were caught, on paper preferably, which the midwife disposed of, usually by gently dropping them into a stream or burying them. Burning was not permitted because the special soul of the child might be present in the birth fluids and should not be harmed. Even today many Chinese women feel they must not worship any gods or visit someone else's house for a month after giving birth.

As civilization progressed, the group became more involved rather than sending the parturient off on her own. Attempts were made to assist difficult labors, which sometimes necessitated leaving the birth structure. Taking the woman into the open and scaring her or tossing her in a blanket held at the corners by four strong individuals were American Indian techniques.

Abnormal births have always been a source of fear, but expectations of physiologic problems did little to influence the site of birth. This attitude differs markedly from the assertion today that birth should take place in an environment equipped to handle any emergency or unusual development. Medical historians seem to agree that most deliveries in primitive societies were normal, with labors of short duration. Women were physically active so their musculature was well developed. Unrefined foods and loose clothing further contributed to their general health. Infection was not a serious problem because contact with sick individuals was usually restricted; instruments and internal examinations were not used. The instinctive suckling of the newborn provided some protection against hemorrhage. Disproportion between the pelvis of the mother and the size of the infant's head may have been rare because so were intermarriages and crossbreeding.

When difficulties such as an abnormal presentation did occur, there were no effective remedies so the environment did not matter. Complicated labors usually resulted in the loss of the child and sometimes the mother as well. Witch doctors, shamans, and priests carried their own paraphernalia and could perform their rituals in any environment, unlike modern physicians who need support equipment and staff to be most effective in a crisis.

POSITIONS AND FURNITURE

An important part of the birth scene is the position of the parturient during the second stage of labor. Historically, almost every conceivable position has been used in childbearing. Associated with this is the furniture used. Most births have taken place on the ground, particularly since most simple huts have no real floors, but as more substantial housing developed, furniture appeared.

Various kinds of chairs, couches, and stools are shown in reliefs of birth scenes from ancient Egypt, Greece, and Rome. The Old Testament also mentions "stools"; scholars claim these were not common but used only by the wealthy or persons of importance. Another interpretation is that the Hebrew word usually translated as birthstool is *ovnayim,* which means "two stones." This may indicate that birth took place outdoors, perhaps in fields where the parturient could lean against stones or brace her feet against them as she pushed.

The upright position, aided by gravity, continued to be used into the Middle Ages as European midwives carried their birthstools from home to home. As men began increasingly to attend lying-in women, the birthstool gave way to special tables or beds. François Mauriceau, considered the best and most famous French accoucheur of the seventeenth century, delivered most of his patients' babies in their own beds at home. Legend claims that Louis XIV promoted the use of beds because he enjoyed watching his mistresses give birth; it was easier to view the scene when the parturient was on a raised platform. In any case, it became fashionable to deliver on a bed and even today home births generally take place on a bed.

By the eighteenth century a great variety of obstetric chairs, couches, tables, and beds were being designed in Europe. Most could be adjusted for a sitting or reclining position, and many had changeable footstops. Flat delivery tables with stirrups, sometimes elaborate contraptions, became more common at the end of the nineteenth century as the number of hospital births began increasing. Critics of the medical establishment have interpreted these gadgets as another example of unnecessary intervention.

Decorum was another aspect of the choice of a birth environment. The mother's bedchamber was considered both more private and more comfortable. Often during the seventeenth and eighteenth centuries the male midwife or barber-surgeon waited in an antechamber while the parturient was attended by females. He would be called into the birth room only if difficulties developed.

Just as today, the economic and social status of a parturient made a difference. Poverty-stricken women could not be as particular as grand ladies. William Smellie, a great teacher of midwifery in eighteenth century London, provided clinical experience for his students by delivering babies in the slums without charge. In fact, part of the fees paid by students was contributed to these unfortunate families.

Particularly during the nineteenth century in Victorian England and in the United States, the male physician was rarely permitted to view the actual birth process. Modesty decreed that at least a sheet be kept over the entire form of the parturient; the male attendant was supposed to rely on his sense of touch as he placed his hands under the cover but kept his eyes elsewhere. These inhibitions had to be overcome before women would willingly go to hospitals and allow themselves to be placed on delivery tables. *Lying-In: A History of Childbirth in America* by Richard W. Wertz and Dorothy C. Wertz[4] includes an excellent discussion of this modesty issue.

WESTERN CIVILIZATIONS

The most important development in the history of lying-in environments has been the recent phenomenon of births moving from homes into hospitals. Hospitals did not appear until Christian times when clerics were encouraged to offer shelter for wayfarers. The earliest health facilities in Europe were actually hospices—church-operated places for the poor and abandoned to die. Some nursing care was provided, but there were no physicians. The little available medical treatment was offered by monks and nuns in their monasteries and convents or by persons whom the community recognized as healers, often women such as midwives who came into the parturient's home.

Hospitals

The prototype of modern hospitals was developed by the Moslems in the early ninth century. During the Dark Ages in Europe, while Christian hospices were often more concerned about the patient's soul than his or her bodily ailments, the Baghdad of Harun al-Rashid and the Thousand and One Nights witnessed the growth of hospitals as places to promote good health, cure diseases, teach, and expand medical knowledge. Libraries, pharmacies, places for prayer, mortuaries, and residence facilities for staff were being integrated. However, throughout the Abbasid Caliphate, which stretched from Spain across north Africa to the borders of China, birth took place at home. Custom and religious teachings would not allow men to view women's bodies.

One of the most famous European hospitals was the Hôtel Dieu in Paris. According to legend it opened about 660 A.D. as a charitable refuge for the poor. By the eighth century there was a special section for maternity cases, but until the late nineteenth century only desperate women sought this environment for their lying-in. Patients who had any family at all were cared for at home, however humble or luxurious.

The significance of hospitals in a history of birth environments before the twentieth century lay in the opportunity they afforded for education and research. By Renaissance times in Europe, hospitals had become part of the growth of cities and a reflection of increasing knowledge and technical developments. Midwives (male and female) received training in them working on charity cases. During the sixteenth century the first printed instructions for midwives appeared, and it finally became economically feasible for people like the French surgeon Ambroise Paré to seek solutions for difficult labor. One interpretation of the history of midwifery at this time asserts that men began to interfere in the birth process as part of their attempts to dominate women.

During the eighteenth century many hospitals were founded. In Dublin in 1745 Bartholomew Mosse opened the Rotunda, a 15-room house with ten beds to serve poor lying-in women, which became famous as a model for obstetric care. The first lying-in ward attached to a British hospital was in Middlesex; in 1747 William Hunter, an anatomy lecturer, served as a male midwife there. Edinburgh became a focal point for the developing science of obstetrics when a lying-in ward was opened as part of the Royal Infirmary in 1756.

A student of William Hunter's, William Shippen, Jr., is usually considered the first professor of midwifery in America. In 1765 he opened a small, private maternity hospital in Philadelphia for women who were always poor, often alone, and "who might otherwise suffer for want of the common necessities on these occasions." A conservative obstetrician, Shippen did not consider home births unsatisfactory, but he believed his lying-in facility essential for teaching purposes. The presence of men at a normal birth was looked upon as an affront to the modesty of the woman in labor, and only desperate females or those with questionable morals would give birth under such circumstances.

Another important institution in the history of childbirth was the Allgemeines Krankenhaus of Vienna, founded by Empress Maria Theresa (mother of Marie Antoinette) about 1763. By the 1840s when Ignaz Semmelweis was proving that puerperal fever was contagious, it had the largest lying-in ward in the world.

Puerperal fever

For a long time childbed fever was a major problem with hospital births. There were epidemics in Europe in 1664 and 1772, with the severest problems occurring in hospitals. In the 1820s Viennese women pleaded not to be taken to the Allgemeines Krankenhaus; they preferred delivering in the streets of the city. The situation persisted until Semmelweis had demonstrated the effectiveness of certain cleaning procedures, Joseph Lister had promoted his antiseptic methods, and Pasteur had identified the offending streptococcus. The battle against puerperal fever was the most dramatic episode of nineteenth century obstetrics.

UNITED STATES—TRANSITION

Throughout the 1800s the pattern of centuries continued—the vast majority of births took place at home. In the United States most lying-in institutions were small and located in eastern cities where they served as refuges for poor married women whose home environments were lamentable. Unpleasant side effects of the Industrial Revolution were felt even in obstetrics. After the Civil War when it was recognized that unmarried pregnant women needed care, maternity facilities often considered social rehabilitation a part of their task. Some maternity centers that were connected with medical schools were instrumental in the advancement of knowledge, and the emphasis began to shift from moral uplifting to scientific interest in the process of birth itself.

The big shift of the birth experience into hospitals came in the twentieth century and was most accelerated in the United States. In 1900 less than 5% of all American babies were born in hospitals; the figure increased to 50% by 1940 and to 99% by 1975. The reason stressed publicly for this dramatic change was a growing belief that hospital births were safer for both mother and infant. Specialized facilities and around-the-clock care were particularly important for difficult deliveries. As women had fewer babies, the concern for the health of each individual increased. The women's movement stressed that women were entitled to the best possible care.

Increasing urbanization and improved methods of transportation, especially the automobile, made hospitals accessible to more people. No longer were rural American women excluded from up-to-date care.

Social reasons

Changing mores also played a role in the movement of births to institutional settings. By the end of the nineteenth century it had become fashionable to give birth in a hospital with a trained male physician as opposed to a supposedly igno-rant midwife. Urbanization had separated families so that there were fewer net-works of women relatives and friends to help one another. Servants were less com-mon, and the hospital confinement was viewed as a vacation from the usual chores at home. It seemed easier to remove the physical aspects of birth and the need to clean up afterward out of the home. American hospitals actively fostered the idea that they were pleasant and comfortable places.

The notion of comfort was carried further with the importation of Twilight Sleep from Europe around the First World War. Morphine was injected at the beginning of labor, scopolamine was used as an amnesiac, and ether or chloroform was ad-ministered when the baby entered the birth canal. American physicians did not favor this procedure, although few would have agreed with Charles D. Meigs, a prominent Philadelphia obstetrician of the mid-nineteenth century who wrote that the pain of childbirth was "a desirable, salutary, and conservative manifestation of life force." However, American women wanted less painful deliveries. In 1914 Dr. Eliza Taylor Ransom, a homeopathic physician who had "gone through hell" twice herself, set up her own maternity hospital in Boston and actively advertised and promoted twilight sleep. Upper-class ladies such as Mrs. John Jacob Astor en-dorsed it publicly, and physicians felt obliged to yield to their patients' requests. This seemed to require that birth take place in a hospital, and physicians soon recognized that this procedure made their patients more manageable. It also fit an image of feminine passivity that many advocated in the 1920s and 1930s. It was not until later that mothers and physicians began to understand that anesthetics and drugs could harm infants.

In the 1920s women's magazines advocated hospital births for many of these reasons. Their emphasis on greater cleanliness in institutions as well as their trained personnel appealed to the middle class. The only way for poor urban women, separated from their families, to obtain care was by going to a hospital; midwives who attended births at home were disappearing for a number of reasons.

Government involvement

The federal government became involved as concern for infant and maternal health received public attention in the 1880s. Investigations by the Children's Bu-reau, which was established in 1912, revealed relatively high maternal and infant mortality. As state and federal programs in the health field increased, funds were channeled through hospitals, thus influencing the birth environment.

Some historians have suggested that the medical establishment encouraged this movement of births into hospitals for its own convenience. In reality, the recog-nized shortage of qualified physicians during the first half of this century necessi-tated more efficient use of their time. Although gradually the demands of hospital routines often took priority over the patients' needs for individualized care, this was not the original reason for advocating birth in an institution. The medical establishment became more directly involved after the organization of the American Board of Obstetrics and Gynecology in 1930. One specific purpose was to set criteria for hospitals so that safety could be improved, and as a result maternal and infant mortality statistics improved significantly.

Medical insurance

Since World War II medical insurance has been a major reason for the increase in hospital births. For example, the Frontier Nursing Service began in Kentucky in 1925 and became a model of traditional midwifery, which meant home births. Their mortality record was better than the national average, largely because of their emphasis on prenatal care. However, since 1960 the birth environment has increasingly been the hospital; insurance payments would not be made for home births.

In the 1950s feelings of alienation toward hospitalization began to surface, and in the 1960s vocal, organized opposition grew. Some of the reasons for giving birth in hospitals were questioned; some studies indicated there was greater safety in home births for normal deliveries; comfort was no longer considered more likely to be found in a hospital; with the increased popularity of "natural" or "prepared childbirth," the need for hospital-administered pain killers faded; and feminist critics proclaimed that the hospital environment intensifies manipulation of women by physicians.

EUROPE

The movement of the majority of births into hospitals was most rapid in the United States, but European and other technologically-advanced countries have followed the trend. In 1954 about half the babies in England were born at home; by 1974 only 8% were home births. There are still special schools for domiciliary midwives, but most English midwives are now nurses with postgraduate training in obstetrics. In Denmark hospital deliveries became more fashionable in the 1970s, and the government-encouraged 300-year tradition of independent midwives and home births is fading.

According to Suzanne Arms,[1] the greatest choice of birth environments and attendants is in the Netherlands, which has lower infant mortality than the United States. By 1973 only 40% of all births there took place at home. All combinations of location (hospital, clinic, or home) and attendant (obstetrician, family physician, or midwife) are covered by the national health insurance plan. Birth is considered a normal although strenuous process. Emphasis is on safety, economy, and making the experience as pleasant as possible.

UNDERDEVELOPED AREAS

In underdeveloped areas of the world childbirth is too often governed by customs and financial limitations that produce unsuitable environments. Oscar Lewis[3] described childbirth in the village of Tepoztlan, south of Mexico City, in the 1950s. A *petate,* or curtain, was hung in front of the mother's bed with another on the floor beside her bed where she actually gave birth. The midwife would massage her abdomen with heated oils, and sometimes certain herbs were burned in a clay pot to help the baby emerge more easily. Warm drinks for the mother and wrapping her in a blanket were considered beneficial. After the third stage, the mother's abdomen was bound with a sash, clean clothing was wrapped around her, and she was raised to her bed. The midwife would then remove all soiled items and bathe the baby. The tradition was that the mother stayed behind her curtain in her home for at least 8 days and, if economically possible, took 40 days of bed rest with no duties and repeated sweatbaths.

As governments become more effective and economic conditions improve, increased attention is being focused on maternal and child health. The Mexican government in the 1970s was actively attempting to raise the standards for traditional birth attendants (TBAs) and improve the quality of medical care. One responsibility of the TBA, which the World Health Organization (WHO) is encouraging, is the cleanliness of the birth site (wherever it may be).

In the People's Republic of China one of the first health measures taken by the communists was the establishment of "maternity stations." One reason was to make care more efficient, thus using labor more productively. Except in very remote areas, most deliveries have been moved out of homes and into hospitals or clinics, under the supervision of paramedics.

FUTURE

As the decade of the 1980s begins, women still use an enormous variety of birth environments. The United States has witnessed a phenomenal movement into hospitals, where the majority of American babies are born despite the growing number of alternatives and organizations promoting them. In Europe and other industrialized regions the trend continues to follow the American example, and more infants are delivered in clinics or hospitals. Worldwide, most births are *not* in institutions, but, where Western, scientific methods are becoming known, the preference for a hospital environment and a trained physician is increasing.

Although many American institutions have become large and impersonal, the reality is that medical institutions will continue to play an important role in the future of childbearing.

REFERENCES

1. Arms, S.: Immaculate deception: a new look at women and childbirth in America, Boston, 1975, Houghton Mifflin.
2. Graham, H.: Eternal Eve: the history of gynaecology and obstetrics, Garden City, N.Y., 1951, Doubleday.
3. Lewis, O.: Tepoztlan—village in Mexico, New York, 1960, Holt, Rinehart & Winston.
4. Wertz, R. W., and Wertz, D. C.: Lying-in, a history of childbirth in America, New York, 1977, The Free Press Division of Macmillan.

SUGGESTED READINGS

Breckinridge, M.: Wide neighborhoods: a story of the Frontier Nursing Service, New York, 1952, Harper & Bros.

Cianfrani, T: A short history of obstetrics and gynecology, Springfield, Ill. 1960, Charles C Thomas, Publisher.

Cutter, I. S., and Viets, H. R.: A history of midwifery, Philadelphia, 1964, W. B. Saunders Co.

Ehrenreich, B., and English, D.: Witches, midwives and nurses—a history of women healers, Old Westbury, N.Y., 1973, The Feminist Press.

Findley, P.: Priests of Lucina: the story of obstetrics, Boston, 1939, Little, Brown & Co.

Radcliffe, W.: Milestones in midwifery, Bristol, England, 1967, John Wright & Sons.

Reed, E.: Woman's evolution: from matriarchal clan to patriarchal family, New York, 1975, Pathfinder Press.

Speert, H.: Iconographia gyniatrica, a pictorial history of gynecology and obstetrics, Philadelphia, 1973, F.A. Davis Co.

Wolf, M., and Witke, R., editors: Women in Chinese society, Stanford, Calif., 1975, Stanford University Press.

CHAPTER 2

The Manchester experience

Whatever death is, birth is the opposite.
Pierre Vellay

In the joint position statement published by the Interprofessional Task Force on Health Care of Women and Children in 1978, it was recommended that hospitals offer the option of using a "birthing room," a combination labor and delivery room, rather than a standard delivery room, which resembles a surgical facility. At the time of this position statement, the labor-delivery rooms at Manchester Memorial Hospital had been in successful operation for more than 10 years.

PHILOSOPHY

These fully equipped labor-delivery rooms (or birthing rooms) were developed on the premise that childbirth is basically a normal physiologic event and a powerful emotional experience. However, since childbirth is occasionally abnormal, these birthing rooms provide an appropriate milieu in which many different support systems are synthesized to reduce the risks, minimize intervention, and maximize the joy of childbirth—all within the hospital setting.

BEGINNINGS

The Manchester experience began with my (P.S.) consciousness-raising while in private practice in Manchester, Connecticut. During my first 7 years of practice I delivered more than 2000 babies by routinely medicating and anesthetizing the mothers and excluding the fathers from the birth. My change from conventional, stereotyped routines to individualized, humanistic practice was a slow, painful learning process.

By 1967, the women's movement had become a major social force in this country. Since my obstetric practice is devoted to the health of women and their babies, I listened to the spokespeople and found that what they said made sense.

Women's demands to have control over their reproductive processes resulted in legislation granting them the right to limit their families. At the same time women became better informed about the birth process than ever before and thus less willing to be patronized by obstetricians. The image of the physician as "all-knowing," dealing with a passive, uninformed woman, was fast becoming history.

Couples were planning their families and attending classes in prenatal and post-natal care. A growing awareness of the undesirable side effects of many substances, coupled with a reawakening interest in physical fitness, led many couples to seek a more "natural" way to give birth. National organizations, such as the American Society for Psychoprophylaxis in Obstetrics (ASPO) and the International Child-birth Education Association (ICEA), were telling parents about methods of pre-pared childbirth. In prenatal classes expectant mothers were learning how to cope with each step of labor and delivery. The La Leche League had become a national spokesgroup for the return to breastfeeding. In addition to the nutritional benefits of breast feeding, La Leche mothers were taught that a nursing baby tends to be held more by the mother and therefore may be psychologically closer to her. Thus childbirth was being demystified.

Since I was uninformed about prepared childbirth techniques, I began to read books written by Dr. Grantly Dick-Read of England, Dr. Fernand Lamaze and Dr. Pierre Vellay of France, Dr. Chabon and Dr. Bradley of the United States, and Dr. Velvovsky of the Soviet Union. They advocated delivering babies using little or no medication, just relaxation and breathing techniques for coping with the pain of labor.

The topics covered in the books included midwives, European hospital beds that served as both labor and delivery beds, prenatal education, the husbands' presence throughout labor and birth, and monitrices, nurses who teach prenatal classes and support the couple through labor and delivery. None of this had been included in my medical school curriculum, and I began to wonder if there might be a better way.

By spring of 1967 my curiosity was sufficiently aroused for my wife and I to travel to Paris to seek that "better way." When we arrived, I immediately con-tacted Dr. Pierre Vellay, an obstetrician carrying on the practice of Dr. Lamaze, who had died 10 years before. At the Belvedere Hospital in Paris I had an experi-ence that profoundly changed my professional career. The approach to childbirth I witnessed that night differed drastically from birth as I had experienced it in the United States.

There were two women in labor with their first babies. Each woman was in a room of her own on a comfortable labor-delivery bed, adaptable to her needs and yet easily converted into delivery position when she was ready to give birth. Man-aging labor and delivery as a continuum seemed totally logical, and yet in the United States I had been trained to manage these two aspects of childbirth as if they were separate entities.

At the Belvedere Hospital, although encouraged by her husband, each woman was primarily supported by a monitrice who had been her prenatal instructor in the psychoprophylactic method. These monitrices were both the woman's and the man's primary support. The monitrices remained close to the women, reminding them how to relax, breathe, and concentrate. When delivery was imminent, mother, monitrice, father, and physician worked together as a team. The couples gave birth in a way that was synchronous and joyous, without a need for the intrusive obstetrics I was accustomed to practicing in the United States.

Each woman I observed was in active labor, experiencing strong uterine contractions but handling them by concentrating, breathing over the peak of the contractions, and then resting well between them. When stage two approached, each woman consciously and effectively pushed to expel her baby. Although I had been in practice for 7 years and completed my residency in a hospital with a census of 6000 births a year, I had never seen such effective pushing techniques. As each woman pushed and relaxed her perineum at the same time, the babies' heads made visible progress. One woman was able to bring the baby's head down to a delivery position in approximately six contractions.

The atmosphere in these combined labor-birth rooms was one of support and patience. Dr. Vellay, monitrice, mother, and father rested between contractions and waited patiently for the next one to begin.

Although Dr. Vellay did not perform an episiotomy that evening, it was necessary to repair small bilateral periurethral lacerations after each birth. Because it is possible that with a small episiotomy they could have avoided these lacerations, I have emphasized individualizing decision making regarding episiotomies.

The first baby born that night was pink and cried lustily. As the baby was given to the mother to hold immediately after birth, she radiated a glow of fulfillment that her husband shared. The baby was not taken to the nursery but was weighed and examined in the labor-delivery room. The parents were thus able to become acquainted with, fondle, and nurse the baby, engaging in the attachment activities of the immediate postpartum period.

My conversion to the practice of humanized obstetrics had begun. In addition to attending as many births with Dr. Vellay as possible, I enrolled in a psychoprophylactic course. The teacher, Mme. Rennert, individually instructed each woman in relaxation techniques, emphasizing active participation of the mind throughout the childbirth experience. They were taught a mental process in which the mind is occupied with the thought of relaxing each muscle. Special breathing patterns, conditioning exercises, and a series of conditioned responses were learned so that the woman in labor could respond to contractions by relaxing muscles in parts of her body and breathing in prescribed manner. Concentrating on a focal point in

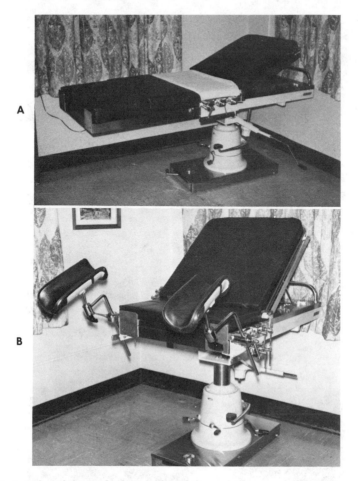

Fig. 2-1. **A,** Labor-delivery bed. **B,** Labor-delivery bed converted to delivery position.

the room during the contractions was also suggested to keep her mind fully occupied.

In review, the essential features of the French management of labor and birth that differed fundamentally from the American technique were (1) the private labor-delivery room within which the total experience took place; (2) a functional labor-delivery bed that was used during both labor and birth; this bed, with no side rails or restraints, was easily converted to the delivery position when the lower half was pushed into the upper half (Fig. 2-1); this created a larger area at the foot

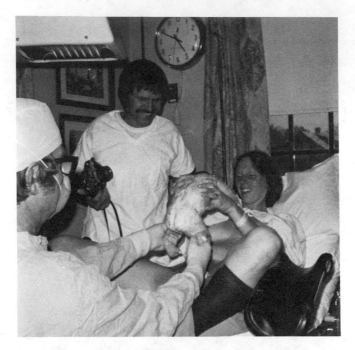

Fig. 2-2. A couple active in their child's birth.

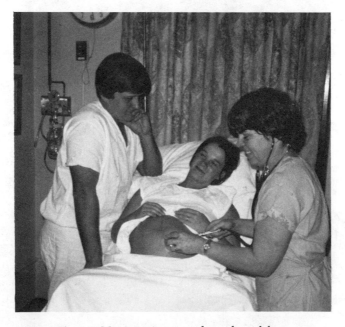

Fig. 2-3. Monitrice support throughout labor.

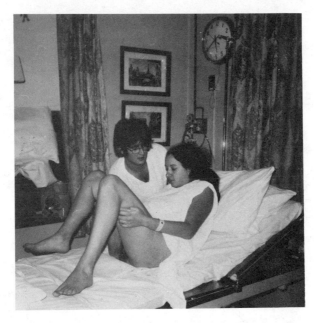

Fig. 2-4. A couple about to become parents . . . together.

of the bed for maneuverability during the delivery; (3) the preparation, both physical and emotional, of the woman herself, enabling her to take an active part in her
labor; (4) the one-to-one continuous support by the monitrice throughout labor and
delivery; and (5) the presence of the husband, offering emotional security and
warmth.

RETURNING HOME

With the guidance and experience that I received from Dr. Vellay and his staff
it appeared to me that I had found a better way for women to give birth. However,
I recognized that it would not be implemented readily in my community, since
historically American medicine has been slow to accept cross-cultural influences.

The American obstetric situation as it existed when I returned from France was
negative and unattractive to me. Mothers were still heavily medicated and passive,
and fathers were denied participation in labor and birth. Babies were often depressed and in need of resuscitation. This was in marked contrast to the exciting
experiences in Paris where the mother and father were actively involved in the
birth experience, using minimal or no medication or anesthesia.

I immediately began trying to interest women who were going to deliver soon

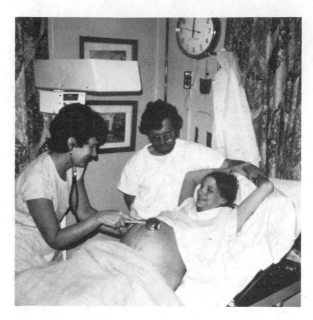

Fig. 2-5. Sandy Eckstrom in her role as fetal monitrice.

in learning about prepared childbirth through books, since there were no child-birth educators available in northern Connecticut at that time. My goal was to find women who wanted to prepare for an active role in their labors and births. The first person who helped me reach that goal was a nurse named Sandra Eckstrom. She was thrilled with the birth of her first baby and is still teaching in our prepared childbirth program today.

Nevertheless, the resistance I met from my senior partner and colleagues was formidable. In fact, during the summer of 1967 the only progress I was able to see was with patients and potential instructors. During this discouraging summer, pressure to change was exerted on the medical community by a consumer group identified by the acronym CALM (Connecticut Association for the Lamaze Method). This organization has done much to foster prepared childbirth and to make southern Connecticut today progressive in terms of the psychoprophylactic method. Shortly after this an organization called PACE (Parents Association for Childbirth Education) was formed in Hartford and began agitating for a change in maternity attitudes and policies.

Another step forward occurred when an office nurse, Billie Carlson, traveled to New York City to become the first certified Lamaze instructor north of Stamford, Connecticut.

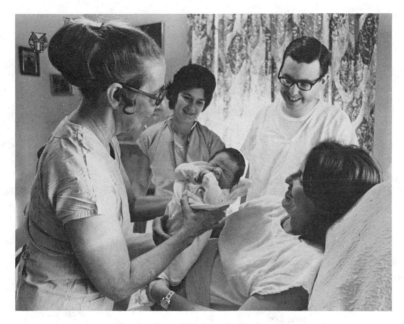

Fig. 2-6. Billie Carlson handing baby to a new mother.

During this time the medical community resisted change in every possible way. When my proposal that our hospital obstetrics department sponsor classes of the Lamaze type was coldly received, we decided the only answer was to have private instructors teach Lamaze in their homes or outside the hospital. Our program at Manchester is still based on this plan, and the theme of hominess, warmth, and congeniality is a binding thread.

In October, 1967, a new partner, John Wheeler, joined our practice. He proved to be a strong proponent of the major changes required to introduce an appropriate, effective, and complete prepared childbirth program in our hospital.

In December, 1968, after $1^{1}/_{2}$ years of frustration with our inability to practice obstetrics as we felt we had the right, with prepared husbands in the delivery room, we took our case to the hospital grievance committee.

It was their opinion, after hearing both sides, that our hospital should permit husbands to remain with their wives in the delivery room if the physician requested it. They further recommended that the hospital develop facilities so that the husband and and wife could stay together through labor and delivery. I proposed that Dr. Wheeler and I perform deliveries in the labor room, but first it would have to be equipped as a first-class labor-delivery room, which involved

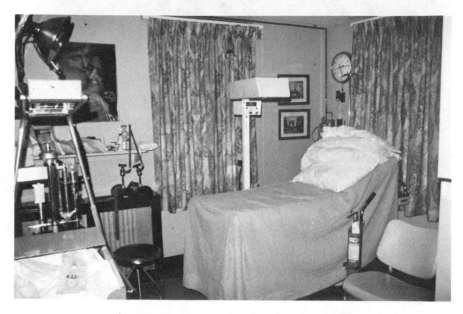

Fig. 2-7. First birth room at Manchester Memorial Hospital.

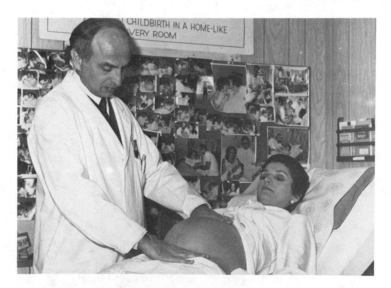

Fig. 2-8. Dr. Wheeler with Cecelia Hasel in office examining room.

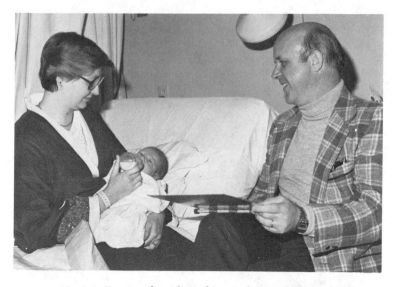

Fig. 2-9. Dr. Smith with Barbara Stabile and Michael.

acquisition of a labor-delivery bed and installation of appropriate ancillary equipment, such as shelving, suction, oxygen, and a Kreiselman incubator.

The administration and our colleagues agreed to this. However, it was further stipulated that the obstetric staff nurses were already too busy in the regular labor and delivery area and that, therefore, we would have to supply our own nurses for this separate labor-delivery room. What at first seemed to be a hardship turned out to be the greatest single asset of our program, since it enabled us to introduce the concept of the monitrice. One-to-one, uninterrupted support of the highly motivated and sympathetic monitrice has helped ensure the success of our program.

In 1969, our senior partner left the practice, and the following year our practice and program received another major boost when Dr. Samuel G. Smith joined Dr. Wheeler and me. Dr. Smith has always been an active advocate of conscious childbirth and fit into our practice like a hand in a glove.

THE CHILDBEARING FAMILY

Evidence of our program's popularity is that Manchester Memorial Hospital, which serves a population of about 100,000, has managed to increase its births over the past several years in a state with the lowest birthrate in the country. More than 4000 women have given birth in our labor-delivery rooms, including several who traveled from New York, Massachusetts, and Kentucky.

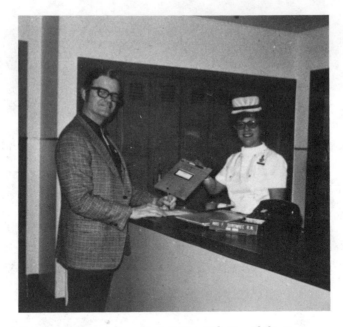

Fig. 2-10. Frances Surowiec, R.N., with Dr. Philip Sumner.

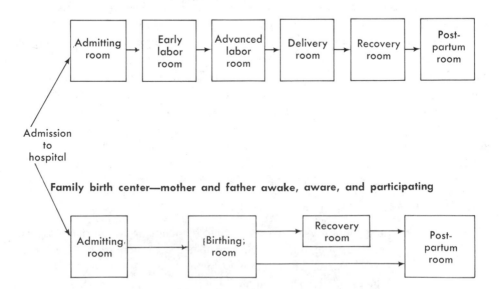

Fig. 2-11. Traditional vs. birthing room flow chart.

At Manchester Hospital, a woman can choose the way her individual labor and delivery will be handled. If she wants to labor and deliver in one place, she can; she may remain awake, aware, and participatory throughout; her husband may or may not be present, as the couple chooses. If she has taken Lamaze classes, she can decide to have a monitrice in attendance or not; or she can choose a traditional delivery (Fig. 2-11). Fortunately, most women opt to take an active rather than a passive role in the birth of their babies.

Screening criteria

Although the majority who use the birthing rooms are well prepared for child-birth through the Lamaze classes, the program is not restricted to Lamaze-pre-pared women. All candidates for vaginal delivery may use the birth rooms; there are no risk criteria for eligibility. If problems develop, they are managed the same as in a standard delivery room. The safety of either the high-risk or the normal mother is not compromised in any way. Transfer to the standard delivery room is at the discretion of the birth attendant. As confidence in using the birth room builds, transfers become less and less frequent. Most occur when it is necessary to have general anesthesia available. The mother is then transferred to a stretcher and easily wheeled into the regular delivery room only 10 feet away, a procedure no more inconvenient than that to which she is routinely subjected in most maternity units today.

THE BIRTHING ROOM
Labor-delivery bed

Except for the unavailability of general anesthesia, the labor-delivery room (birth room) is in every way a first-class delivery room. Drapes in the windows, pictures on the warmly colored walls and a radio, if desired, create a pleasant atmosphere. A rocking chair is provided for the mother and a comfortable chair for the father. A wide mirror is located at the foot of the bed so both may observe the delivery, and a phone is handy so parents can share the celebration with relatives and friends.

After a fruitless search for an adequate American-made labor-delivery bed, a suitable French model was located and imported. Of excellent workmanship, the bed is comfortable for labor and has seven adjustable positions for back support. Conversion for delivery involves merely placing the woman's legs into the heavily padded leg supports at hip level, pushing the lower half of the bed into the upper half, and wheeling in a splash basin and instrument table. However, if leg supports are not desired, they can simply be used for the woman to prop her legs against. The labor-delivery bed offers a happy contrast to the automatic transfer in the con-ventional maternity unit.

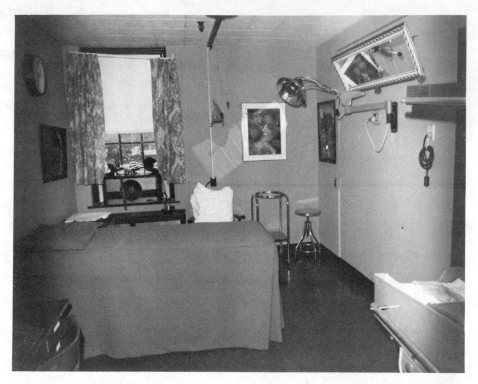

Fig. 2-12. Another birth room in Manchester Memorial Hospital, known as the "Gold Room" because of the warm gold tones used in decorating it.

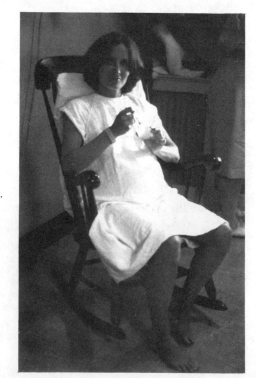

Fig. 2-13. A laboring woman in rocking chair.

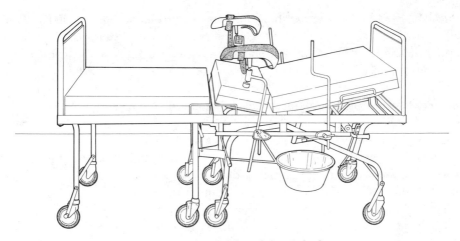

Fig. 2-14. Dutch labor-delivery bed.

Fig. 2-15. Steel's English obstetric table; foot end telescoped under head for forceps delivery.

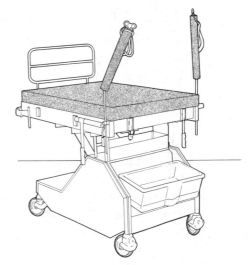

Each of several European countries has its own uniquely designed labor-delivery bed, but they share similarities, including a recognition of the physiologic continuity of the labor-delivery process. The Dutch have a separating bed, the lower half of which can be wheeled out of the room (Fig. 2-14). The woman's legs may then be placed in the stirrups, or the birth attendant, by kneeling, may assist with in-bed delivery without stirrups.

The English labor-delivery bed has pedals and all the instruments for adjustment at the head of the bed to be operated by the anesthesiologist (Fig. 2-15). The much superior French bed is adjustable at the foot or side so that it may be placed against a wall, leaving maximum room for delivery even in a small labor room. It was designed by a Parisian obstetrician, Dr. DeSoubry, 60 years ago and has been clinically tested by three generations of French women and improved. Dr. Pierre Vellay strongly recommended Dr. DeSoubry's lit-table obstetric bed (manufactured in Paris by Pierre Mathieu and Co.) because of its solidity, comfort, and versatility (Fig. 2-16).

The Swedish labor-delivery table can be adjusted to an upright position for delivery. However, again, all the pedals for operating the bed are not readily available for the delivering attendant to use (Fig. 2-17). Recent American designs for labor-delivery beds include the Borning Bed (Fig. 2-18) and birthing beds designed by Stryker Corporation (Fig. 2-19) and Borg-Warner Health Products, Inc. (Fig. 2-20). There are many variations of labor-delivery beds in use and being developed, but all of them have in common the recognition that childbirth is an ongoing experience.

The advantages of a labor-delivery bed may be summarized as follows:

1. The mother is able to concentrate on pushing her baby out without expending energy moving to a stretcher and then moving again to the delivery table.
2. The mother's vital signs may be taken continuously if necessary, and the fetal monitor may remain in place until the baby is born.
3. The father is able to provide continuous support and does not have to be redirected to the new location.
4. If rapid delivery is necessary, the woman's legs may be placed in the leg supports and the baby born quickly without time being wasted in transport to a delivery room.
5. The nursing staff no longer has to make decisions on when to move the mother to the delivery room.
6. There is no second room to be set up, so the nurses have ample time to prepare for an in situ delivery.
7. The physician has more complete control over the labor-delivery sequence and is able to provide the family with as simple, dignified, and enjoyable a childbirth experience as is compatible with medical safety while still facilitating optimum bonding.
8. The hospital benefits by more extensive use of the labor rooms, less laundry and equipment involved, and smaller delivery area.
9. It may be possible to reduce costs, since fewer rooms are used. A delivery room is of course still necessary but can be held in reserve for difficult births: twins, breeches, and those necessitating general anesthesia.
10. The public relations of the hospital can benefit by the presentation of this favorable, "progressive," family-oriented program.
11. Forceps application, vacuum extraction, episiotomy, manual removal of the placenta, and other obstetric techniques can be performed safely if and when necessary.

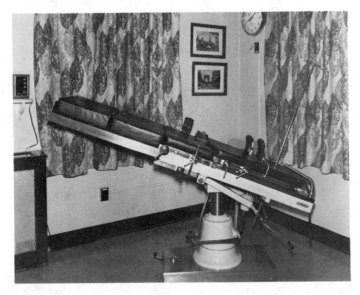

Fig. 2-16. Trendelenburg position obtained rapidly with side handle. Adjustable shoulder and wrist braces secure patient. All controls located at foot or side of bed for ready accessibility; IV pole attachment.

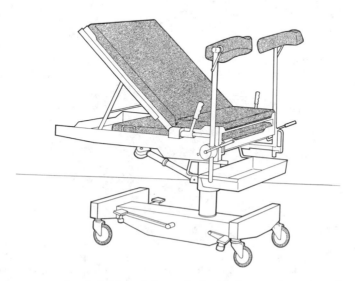

Fig. 2-17. Swedish labor-delivery bed with foot section recessed.

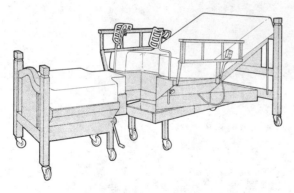

Fig. 2-18. The Borning Bed.

Fig. 2-19. The L'D^{+1} bed designed by Stryker
Corporation.

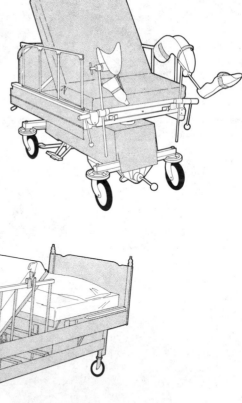

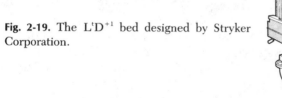

Fig. 2-20. Birthing bed by Borg-Warner Health Products, Inc.

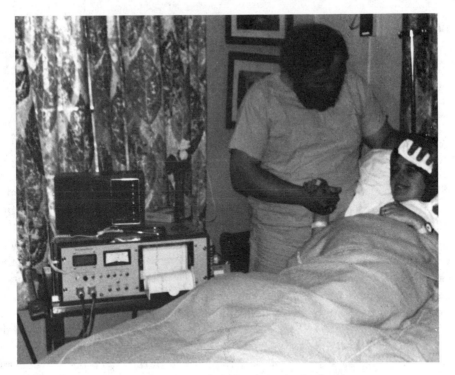

Fig. 2-21. Electronic fetal monitoring in birth room.

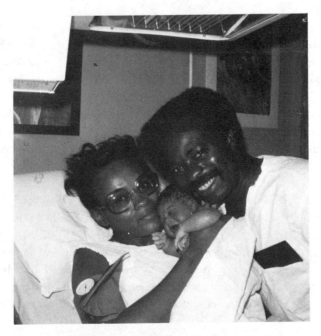

Fig. 2-22. Jessie and Joe Ballenger bonding with their son.

Medication and anesthesia

If pain relief is requested by a mother, a modified paracervical block is uniquely suitable. When given in small divided doses (2.5 ml each of mepivacaine 1% [Carbocaine]) and injected slowly submucosally and well lateral in the vaginal vaults it has an immediate effect. Side effects and systemic absorption are minimal, and fetal bradycardia is rare. The paracervical block has the remarkable capability of decreasing uterine and cervical discomfort, therefore enabling the woman to be conscious and participating in her labor and delivery in a controlled fashion even when not using prepared childbirth techniques.

Since a modified paracervical block is a simple anesthetic given by the obstetrician, the anesthesiologist no longer needs to be in attendance on the maternity floor. The paracervical block is an ideal backup technique for the prepared mother because it in no way changes the premises on which her method of labor is based, i.e., it does not interfere with her ability to concentrate, relax, breathe, move, ambulate, squat, or push in the appropriate fashion. Also, small amounts of the anesthetic can be given just in the area where she is having the discomfort. For example, if the pain is on the left side in her back, the block can be given at just 5 o'clock well lateral to the cervix. If the pain is on the right in the back, the paracervical block is given at 7 to 8 o'clock, which is the area of the right uterosacral ligament. The paracervical block may be given during stage one of labor and repeated if necessary. Although the paracervical block, the pudendal block, and local infiltration are never used routinely, they are available for any mother who may require them.

The need for systemic medication has been greatly reduced by our program's emphasis on prenatal preparation and support during labor. Extremely apprehensive mothers, such as we used to see, are rare. However, occasionally it may be necessary to use small amounts of a tranquilizing drug such as 25 mg meperidine (Demerol) or 25 mg hydroxyzine pamoate (Vistaril). Since participation is stressed, scopolamine is never used. Epidural anesthesia by the obstetrician and/or methoxyflurane (Penthrane) mask is used occasionally, but whenever an anesthetist is required (for spinal, saddle, or general), the mother is transferred to the delivery room.

Staffing

At Manchester, in addition to the regular nursing staff, 14 maternity nurses trained specifically in the Lamaze method of prepared childbirth are available to provide Lamaze-prepared couples with emotional and physical individualized support throughout labor and the immediate postpartum period. By designing a 24-hour call schedule, the monitrices provide a supplementary nursing service, which helps to resolve the constant problem of staffing for peak and overflow periods on

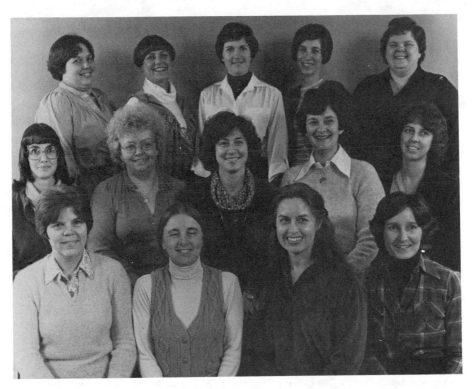

Fig. 2-23. Members of Manchester Monitrice Associates, Inc. Back row, left to right: Sue Moore, Harriet Brooks, Barbara Buus, Gerri Schnobrich, Marilyn Hull. Middle row, left to right: Cathy Cyr (Registrar), Ida Anderson, Judy Rainville, Sandy Eckstrom, Kathy Chmielecki. Front row, left to right: Marcia Memery, Sharon Young, Barbara Soderberg, Betsy Tonkin.

obstetric services. The monitrice is not an employee of the hospital or physician and bills the family directly. Thus her primary responsibility is to the family, and she may in a sense be considered a "patient or family advocate."

These monitrices reinforce the father's role without interference. Eight of them also teach childbirth education classes. The following outline briefly describes the organization of the Manchester Monitrice Associates:

A. Childbirth education division
    1. Eight certified teachers—ASPO
    2. Lamaze method—six classes
    3. Home based—informal
    4. Limited to six couples
    5. Fee
    6. Many teachers are also montrices

B. Monitrice division
  1. Thirteen obstetric RNs trained in the Lamaze method
  2. Provides monitrice coverage in birthing rooms
  3. Ensures continuous one-to-one support throughout labor and delivery
  4. Optional for Lamaze patients
  5. Fee

The Manchester Monitrice Associates have published a manual on the function of the monitrice in a modern prepared childbirth program.* The following description of a monitrice is taken from the manual:

The monitrice is an established and essential part of the psychoprophylactic method in France and other European countries. She provides uninterrupted, one-to-one, sympathetic, and enthusiastic support of the patient throughout labor and delivery, thus minimizing the need for drugs and anesthetics and maximizing the positive experience of childbirth.

She is familiar with the various relaxation, concentration, breathing, and pushing conditioned responses which the patient has learned during her Lamaze training. She makes certain that the husband is coaching properly, and she does not hesitate to reinforce both husband and patient should either begin to falter. To properly fulfill her job, the monitrice should possess certain special personal qualifications. She should be an experienced nurse trained in both obstetric nursing and the Lamaze method, resourceful, assertive, enthusiastic, dedicated, and able to inspire a feeling of confidence and security. She is similar to a private duty nurse in that her one responsibility is to this patient, not the hospital, and therefore the patient is assured of the continuous uninterrupted support (verbal analgesia) and supervision which are essential. Fathers and other support persons are, of course, very helpful and should give the primary support, but they vary greatly in this capability and often both the father and the mother benefit enormously from words and actions of the backup monitrice. Unlike giving a larger dose of Demerol, increasing the support personnel may significantly increase patient comfort without in any way depressing the baby! She also performs routine nursing duties for the patient and is able to auscultate the fetal heart continuously if necessary, thus performing in a sense the role of a humanized, caring, and comforting fetal monitor ("fetal monitrice"). A stethoscope in the hands of an experienced obstetrical nurse is still a most useful instrument. Of course, the fetal monitor may still be used when necessary, but it should never reduce or replace the role of the continuous caring person, and it should always be low profile, inconspicuous, and not imply morbidity.

By being admitted directly to the room where she is going to deliver, the mother is able to develop increasingly strong feelings of security towards the room and the people in it. Just as it is an obsolete concept to routinely transfer the mother to another room for delivery, so it is equally obsolete to have a change of support personnel just as she is entering transition and beginning to push. How often does it happen that a mother will deliver during or shortly after the relief shift, or the night shift, or the day shift has just come on duty? The mother is then subjected to a double setback at a time when she is most in need of support! She must readjust to both a new and often anxiety-producing

---

*The birth of a monitrice, Manchester, Conn., 1977, Manchester Monitrice Associates; available for nominal fee at 31 Bette Dr., Manchester, Conn. 06040.

environment (the austere D.R.) and new personnel who are unacquainted with her labor prior to coming on duty, and who have not established a strong personal interrelationship, which is so important at this time.

Routine staffing of the labor-delivery floor was adequate when women were routinely medicated and anesthetized. Assembly line, mass-production techniques were acceptable since each woman did not require individualized attention. Thus the same number of nurses could manage five or ten mothers equally well. But the "prepared" woman admitted to a private labor-delivery room in early labor requires the individualized ministrations of a monitrice to assure her the continuity of support and nursing services throughout labor, delivery, and the important, sensitive, immediate postpartum period when the emotional "bonding" of the mother, father, and baby is taking place. Having fully shared in the stress, the strain, and the struggle preceding birth, the monitrice is able to fully participate in the meaningful activities and joyful celebration following the delivery.

The monitrice concept is appropriate for all obstetrical patients whether "high or low risk." In fact, since a "high-risk" mother is likely to have greater anxiety, the need for a constant support person is even more important! Unlike the surgical O.R. schedule, which can be drawn up accurately one day in advance, obstetrics is an unpredictable and emergency-type specialty. It is manifestly impossible to predict ahead of time who or how many will be delivering the next day, or on what shift. It is financially unrealistic for the administrator to attempt to staff each shift with sufficient nurses to assure each woman this essential one-to-one support. By definition, the staff nurse relates to the needs of the hospital and not the needs of any one individual patient. No matter how interested or highly motivated a staff nurse may be, she may have to leave the side of a particular woman to help with a new admission, a delivery, or a stat cesarean delivery. Therefore a flexible "on-call" monitrice program to supplement the regular staff nurses is essential to any hospital offering a complete prepared childbirth program since it helps to resolve the constant dilemma of the feast or famine staffing of the maternity unit.

Staff nurse and monitrice each fulfill an essential function—the former performing the many essential hospital duties and the latter meeting the needs of the individual parturient. Teamwork and cooperation are essential to provide optimum patient care. The staff nurse coordinates with the monitrice by admitting the patient and supporting her until the monitrice arrives, by assuming the responsibility for baby management during delivery, and by caring for the patient after transfer to the postpartum area. She also assists the monitrice in event of complications, preparation for cesarean delivery, etc. The transition to the monitrice concept in a hospital can be facilitated by emphasizing the importance of the caring support person and encouraging the staff nurses to participate in the monitrice program, which has its own very special emotional rewards and satisfactions. The dedicated monitrice, supported by equally dedicated staff nurses, is essential to enable the mother and father to experience the miracle of childbirth under optimum conditions of individuality, safety, and dignity.

After-birth celebration

"Celebration" is the theme of birth in the birthing rooms at Manchester Memorial Hospital. When possible, rheostated dim lights are used as the baby emerges, with the mother herself reaching down and lifting her baby to her breast, assisted slightly so the baby does not slip. In almost every instance, the umbilical

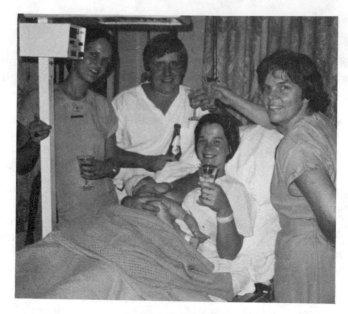

Fig. 2-24. Celebration.

cord is long enough to permit her to determine her infant's sex for herself, and thus immediate bonding is encouraged. Although there is no complete agreement on when to cut the umbilical cord, waiting until pulsations have stopped seems to facilitate delivery of the placenta. By doing episiotomy or laceration repair first, there is additional time for the placenta to spontaneously separate. With proper support, it is still possible to do a gentle manual removal of the placenta, if necessary, without anesthesia.

A radiant warmer allows the baby to make the most painless adjustment from the uterus to the mother's body. The heat panel permits extended skin-to-skin contact between the mother and baby without blankets, since the baby's temperature must be maintained at 97° to 99° F, whereas room temperature is usually 70° to 72° F.

To maximize the parent-infant attachment process, silver nitrate eyedrops for the newborn are withheld for 1 hour. After the parents share the first 60 minutes of their newborn's life in the same labor-delivery room where the birth occurred, the family is transferred together to the newborn nursery, where the baby is given vitamin K and examined thoroughly. If mother and baby are stable with no complications, then by prior arrangement with the pediatrician and obstetrician, they may be transferred directly to a family unit or to the postpartum room for

Text continued on p. 40.

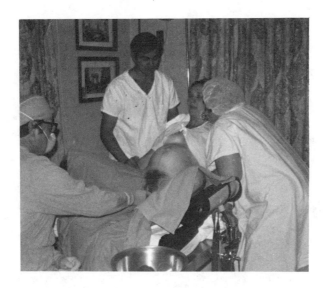

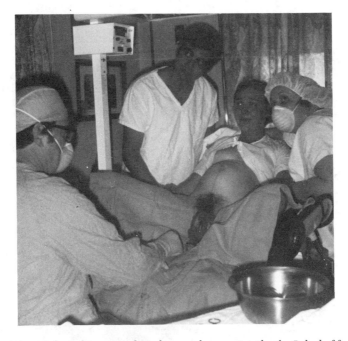

Permission to share this series of 11 photographs was given by the Labadorf family.

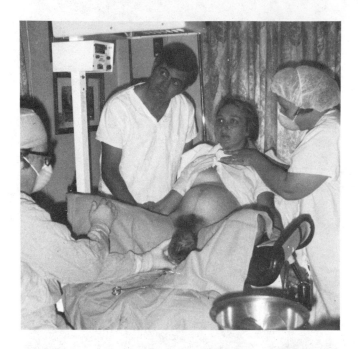

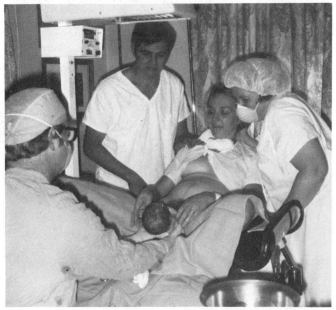

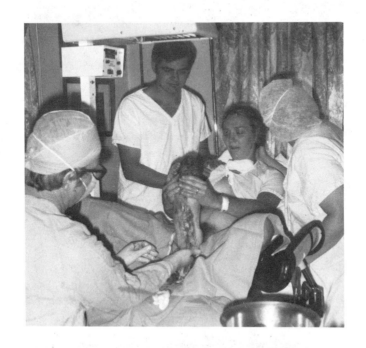

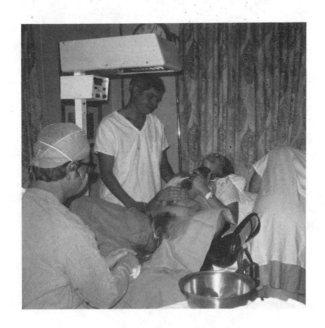

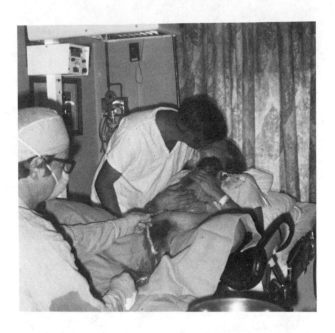

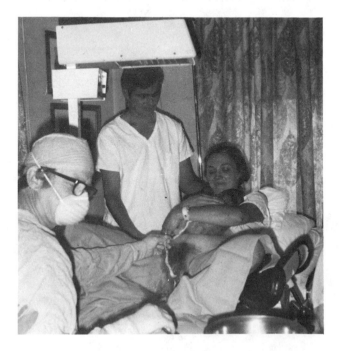

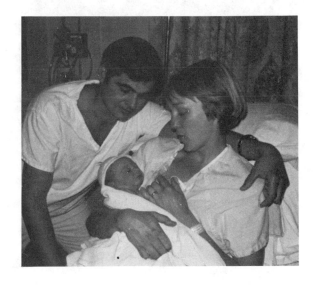

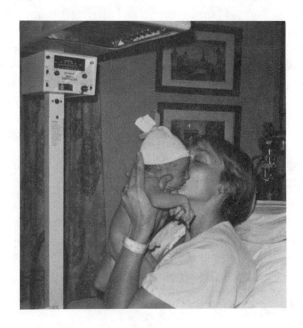

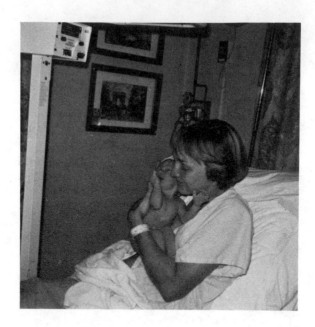

continuous nonseparation. If a problem exists for either the mother or baby, the baby will remain in the newborn nursery, and the mother may be transferred to the recovery room for observation and appropriate treatment.

Breastfeeding, rooming-in, and sibling visitation are encouraged. There is a family visiting room on the postpartum unit where families can be together. In postpartum classes for both father and mother the new parents are encouraged to assume responsibility and gain confidence in their new roles. Early ambulation as well as early discharge are encouraged.

STATISTICS

The transformation of Manchester Memorial Hospital's maternity unit into a family birth center has been a gradual evolution over the past 11 years and is still in progress. In 1969, the first year of the program, 83, or 5%, of the births occurred in the birthing room, whereas in 1978, 731, or 58%, took place in birthing rooms. For the first 5 years of the program all mothers delivering in the birthing room had to have psychoprophylactic preparation and a monitrice. However, in 1974 we opened a second birthing room that was available for any mother, prepared or not, with or without monitrice, who in the opinion of her obstetrician was having a normal labor.

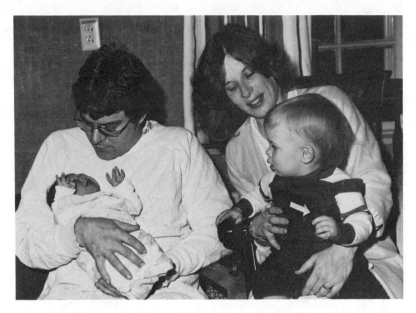

Fig. 2-25. The new family getting acquainted in the sibling visiting room.

Up to this point the entire program had been essentially limited to our three-physician practice. This second room popularized the birthing room concept with the other six obstetricians on the staff, since they now did not have to "buy the entire package" of Lamaze preparation and monitrice support. The second room could also be used for another Lamaze patient with a monitrice if two were in labor at the same time. The room was then managed by the maternity staff nurses, which gave them as well as the other obstetricians the opportunity to become familiar with and recognize the advantages of birthing rooms. Thus in the first year of the second birthing room only 53 mothers (4%) had the benefit of that room without monitrice, whereas in 1978 it was the site of 341, or 27%, of all our births. Each year there has been a gradual increase in the acceptance of Lamaze preparation with or without monitrice by the other obstetricians (Fig. 2-26).

Because of the increasing demand, we later opened a third birthing room as birthing rooms are now the primary place for deliveries in our maternity unit.

Since the first monitrice-attended birth in 1969 the Manchester Monitrice Associates have maintained thorough records of each Lamaze birth with monitrice support in the *Lamaze Log*. Although there has been a total of 4221 deliveries in the birthing rooms in the past 10 years, Tables 1 to 4 and accompanying data are limited to those 2830 births by couples prepared in the psychoprophylactic method and attended in the birthing room by monitrices.

From April, 1969, to June, 1979, 1472 (52%) nulliparous and 1358 (48%) mul-

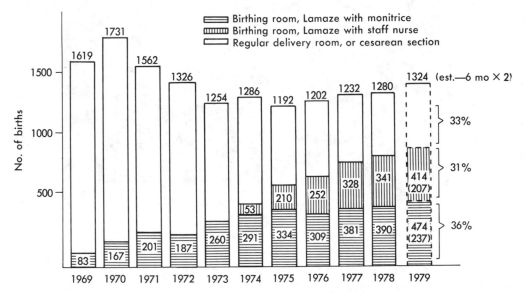

Fig. 2-26. Births at Manchester Memorial Hospital, 1969 to 1979.

Table 1. Nulliparas delivering in place (1290/1472; 88%)

Conditions	Number of women	Percent (%)
Spontaneous	850	66
Vacuum assist*	37	3
Forceps	374	29
Breech	15	1
Twins	14	1

*Represents 2 years' use (1977 to 1979).

Table 2. Multiparas delivering in place (1316/1358; 97%)

Conditions	Number of women	Percent (%)
Spontaneous	1235	94
Vacuum assist*	6	0.5
Forceps	54	4
Breech	12	1
Twins	9	0.5

*Represents 2 years' use (1977 to 1979).

Table 3. Anesthesia used for nulliparas (1290) in birthing room

	Number of women	Percent* (%)	Apgar	
			1 minute	5 minutes
During labor				
Medication	181	14		
Paracervical block	830	64		
None	361	28		
During delivery				
Pudendal block	558	43	8.4	9.0
Local anesthesia	732	57	8.5	9.4
or none				

*Some women received both medication and paracervical block.

Table 4. Anesthesia used for multiparas (1316) in birthing room

	Number of women	Percent* (%)	Apgar	
			1 minute	5 minutes
During labor				
Medication	81	6		
Paracervical block	490	37		
None	814	62		
During delivery				
Pudendal block	302	23	8.6	9.3
Local anesthesia	1014	77	8.7	9.3
or none				

*Some women received both medication and paracervical block.

tiparous women labored and gave birth in the birthing rooms with monitrice. Since in general nulliparas present the obstetrician with the greatest challenges, our program was subjected to rigorous testing from the start. Although it would have been possible to limit the room to multiparas until we gained greater confidence with the program, we believed that it was better to individualize the management of each mother from the very beginning. Even today, "individualize" is the single word that most accurately describes our program.

Roughly only one multipara in 20 had to be transferred from the birthing room to either the regular delivery room or operating room (Table 2). Only 56 (3.8%) nulliparas and 8 (0.6%) multiparas were transferred to the regular delivery room, the primary indication being the need to have general anesthesia available, though not necessarily used. Breech presentation and spinal anesthesia were other of the more common indications for a transfer. Systemic medication is seldom used in the program; total incidence of general anesthesia is 1% and that of spinal 0.5%. Anxiety is primarily managed more fundamentally through prenatal preparation and emotional support. The number of patients transferred and reasons are as follows:

1. General anesthesia available—28
2. Breech delivery—16
3. Midforceps—3
4. Face presentation—2
5. Spinal anesthesia—12
6. Brow—1
7. Scanzoni—1
8. Fetal distress, full dilatation—1

To relieve pain when necessary, 830 (64%) nulliparas and 490 (37%) multiparas had modified paracervical block anesthesia by submucosal technique described earlier. Although pudendal block tends to suppress the pushing reflex, if the mother requests it, it is given.

Maternal complications have been minimal and are managed in the appropriate manner. Fifteen mothers have required transfer to the regular delivery room for general anesthesia during the immediate postpartum period for retained placenta, with two other transfers necessary for laceration of the birth canal, and one for episiotomy hematoma.

A breakdown of the incidence and causes for both fetal and maternal complications follows:

A. Fetal—64/2830 = 2.3%
   1. Stillborn—4
   2. Aspiration pneumonitis—8

    3. Small for dates—33
    4. Depressed Apgar—17
    5. Skull fracture—1
    6. Meningomyelocele—1
B. Maternal—69/2830 = 2.4%
    1. Preeclampsia—10
    2. Premature rupture of membranes—14
    3. Ulcerative colitis—2
    4. Postpartum pneumonia—2
    5. Postpartum bleeding—8
    6. Abruptio placentae—2
    7. Placenta previa—3
    8. Transfer to delivery room post partum for:
        a. Lacerations—2
        b. Retained placenta—15
        c. Episiotomy hematoma—1
    9. Late postpartum hemorrhage—1

There were four stillbirths in the birthing room from 1969 to 1979. This is the statistic that concerns obstetricians the most and drives them to all manner of manipulation and intervention. Yet, we must recognize that although it is important to keep this figure to a minimum, it can never be entirely eliminated. Sometimes by too vigorous intervention we create more problems than we solve.

Analysis of the four stillbirths reveals that one mother was admitted with a questionable fetal heart condition. When an electronic fetal monitor was applied and a confusing pattern obtained, the mother underwent an immediate cesarean delivery of a stillborn. The second mother had a sudden complete placental abruption during the later phases of stage one. The third had deep variable decelerations on the fetal monitor during stage two, although these were thought to be within normal range. The fourth fetus apparently had a good fetal heart condition until 5 minutes before birth but was delivered dead, probably due to sudden cord compression. No autopsies were performed in any of the cases, so internal congenital abnormalities cannot be ruled out. Although the entire goal of our program is to enable couples to have a healthy baby in a dignified and meaningful manner, no such result can be guaranteed. For this reason we feel that, although it is entirely appropriate to celebrate the birth of a healthy baby, it is equally appropriate to grieve along with the parents when tragedy strikes. They understand and appreciate this and it serves to strengthen the physician-parent relationship.

During these 10 years a total of 122 cesarean births (8.4%) were performed on nulliparas and 38 (2.8%) were performed on multiparas; this gives a total primary

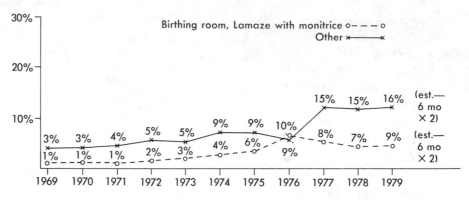

Fig. 2-27. Primary cesarean delivery rates at Manchester Memorial Hospital, 1969 to 1979.

cesarean rate of 160/2830, or 5.7%. The following list enumerates the numbers and indications for the cesarean births:

1. Cephalopelvic disproportion—65
2. Fetal distress—31
3. Breech—23
4. Uterine dystocia—22
5. Prolapsed cord—5
6. Twins—5
7. Transverse lie—3
8. Face—2
9. Placenta previa—2
10. Toxemia—1
11. Intrauterine death prior to labor—1

In the past 5 years we have witnessed, along with the rest of the country, a gradual increase in the primary cesarean rate from 3% in 1973 to 7% in 1978 (Fig. 2-27). However, in comparing the cesarean rate of these Lamaze-prepared mothers with monitrice support to all other primary cesareans performed at our hospital, even allowing for the favorable nutritional and motivational factors, the rate is lower. In 1978, for example, the program for non-Lamaze mothers without a monitrice had a rate of 15% as compared with the Lamaze-montrice program's rate of 7%.

SUMMARY

Childbirth is usually a normal physiologic event and a creative and powerful emotional experience. The aesthetics of birth must be recognized and allowed full expression. Assembly line facilities and routine policies appropriate for the passive woman of 20 years ago are not appropriate for the prepared, participating parents of today. Regimented and disrupted childbirth is impersonal and dehumanizing and has created an austere environment, disenchantment with hospital delivery, and a rapidly growing home birth movement. Hospitals' increasing preoccupation with technology and high-risk pregnancies complicates and confuses childbirth management, increases anxiety, and undermines confidence in the normal processes of labor.

To provide both safety and emotional fulfillment for each birth, hospitals must offer a more joyous model of childbirth, stressing human support in an environment that encourages confidence and patience, emphasizes the art as well as the science of birth, restores faith in the natural mechanism of labor, and thus is more conducive to successful vaginal delivery. Individualization of management of each woman in labor whether healthy or high risk is necessary.

SUGGESTED READING

Interprofessional Task Force on Health Care of Women and Children: Joint position statement on the development of family-centered maternity/newborn care in hospitals, Chicago, June, 1978.

CHAPTER 3

Interviews with families

At the core of the Manchester experience are couples taking an active and meaningful part in childbirth. When developing any facilities for birth, dialogues with families can provide professionals with valuable information to apply the Manchester experience in their own settings. We realize that people tend to remember the good things and forget the unpleasant. However, that realization in itself is why we have given so much space in this book to what "birth memories" people have.

These interviews are not an attempt to measure feelings of satisfaction scientifically, using a control group. Nor are we proposing that these successful birth experiences indicate the discovery of a panacea for all the troubles of today's families. We are simply relating "birth memories" that are representative of those couples who have given birth in the Manchester birth rooms, memories that influence how they feel about themselves as individuals, family members, mates, lovers, and parents.

The couples were not interviewed immediately after giving birth, but instead related their "birth memories" at various times between 5 days and 7 months post partum. Ten of the couples had Lamaze preparation and the support of a monitrice. One couple attended Lamaze classes but chose not to have a monitrice present. Another attended the two prepared childbirth classes at the hospital, and the final couple interviewed had no preparation or special support. We have enlarged on key concepts disclosed in these interviews to provide more information on important aspects of care.

FRED AND SUZANNE STEINHAGEN

Susan Jane was born 10 weeks before this interview. Her sister was $2^{1}/_{2}$ years old. This time, labor began at 2 A.M. for Fred and Sue Steinhagen and moved quickly to delivery about 7 hours later.

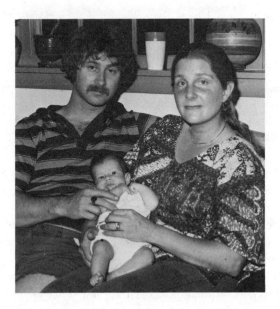

Fred: I think I was much more involved this time. Everything was much more relaxed in the birthing room. The whole time I felt I was right where I should have been. I think the last time I didn't do as much because the fetal monitor was there. Sue couldn't get up, and she couldn't do anything because the fetal monitor prevented it. Since she couldn't move, I couldn't really do anything more than time contractions for her. I really felt that I was just standing around watching the machine. This time I felt like I was involved really because I could participate in what was going on. I was with her the whole time. The monitrice brought me a cup of coffee and I drank it right there in the birth room. We weren't separated even for a minute. I liked this birth better than last time. For one thing, we had the mirror. We didn't have the mirror last time. It was nice for Suzanne, and even for me, because I could see real well from where I was standing.

Suzanne: Everything was so much under control this time. We saw every single detail of her being born. It was wonderful. The other thing I think, for me anyway, was that since this was going to be our last child, I didn't want to miss any of it. That made me zero in even more on everything.

Benefits of father participation

Fred's involvement in this birth experience illustrates how active participation by the father can lead to increased self-esteem for both partners. This couple felt so good about themselves after their experience that they discussed "doing it without help."

>   **Suzanne:** We really could have done it without the doctor. Isn't that terrible? Really though, that's my honest opinion. Even though you need the doctor there, well, really doctors are beginning to feel this way, too, that *you're* the one that's really delivering *your* baby. They are there in case something goes wrong and that really is the role of the doctor now with a program like this. His role is more seeing that you're doing OK each month. That really is almost more important than the delivery, and then to see that everything is going OK in labor, of course.

In investigating the role of husbands in labor and birth, Tanzer[34] compared groups in which the husband was present or absent at birth. The results of this study indicate that the effect on the wives was positive and highly desirable when their husbands were present during the birth. In fact, all women who reported a rapturous or peak experience during birth had their husbands present in the delivery room. In addition, these women experienced increased self-esteem.

Tanzer[34] also found that husbands expressed positive feelings about being actively involved in the birth process, potentially adding a rich dimension to the couple's relationship and ultimately increasing their sense of family.

DENNIS AND JUDY REITER

Dennis and Judy Reiter were interviewed $4\frac{1}{2}$ months after their first child, Geoffrey, was born in a birth room at Manchester Memorial Hospital. Both Dennis and Judy had participated in Lamaze classes as part of their preparation for birth and had also toured the hospital maternity unit prior to labor. Approximately 12 hours after labor began, and with uterine contractions coming every 5 minutes, the Reiters left for the hospital.

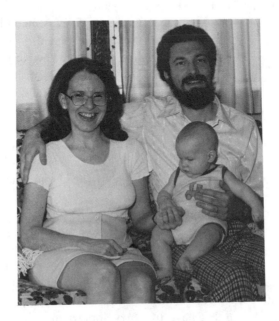

> **Dennis:** We called our neighbors next door to let them know that we were going in and they said, "You know, you don't sound very nervous or scared." And I said, "We're not. We're on an adventure. We're sort of excited." I think that our training had an awful lot to do with it, because basically we had been faithful in doing the exercises, and we know what was going on. So it wasn't as if we were walking into something not knowing 80% of what was going to happen; this made it much easier for us.

Controlled excitement

A feeling of controlled excitement is commonly reported by people who have prepared during pregnancy for coping with labor and birth. In a study by Klusman[17] published in 1975, measures of fear and anxiety were taken before and after classes in preparation for birth for 42 primiparas in the third trimester of pregnancy. Only the childbirth education course (Lamaze method) succeeded in reducing the general anxiety level. It was concluded that childbirth education can reduce fear and anxiety, and that pain perception is enhanced by high anxiety.

Although a direct and linear relationship between maternal anxiety and length of labor has not been proven, Lederman, Lederman, and colleagues[19] studied 32 normal labors to determine the relationship between anxiety, uterine contractility, and plasma catecholamines. Their data indicate that anxiety is correlated with plasma epinephrine. These higher epinephrine levels are correlated with decreased uterine contractility and increased length of labor.

It is encouraging to know that anxiety in pregnancy is modifible. In addition to the study by Klusman,[17] this has been reported by Standley and associates[33] in a longitudinal study of 73 primigravid women and their newborn infants. According to this study, "preparation for childbirth in the form of instructional classes seems to provide the expectant mother with skills of physiologic and/or psychological coping, which combat anxiety."

According to the Reiters, the birth room environment also contributed to the reduction of their anxiety.

Judy: It was in effect like being at home. It is more like a bedroom—homey, so it puts you more at ease. There's not a lot of equipment around and that sort of thing.

Dennis: You didn't get as much of a feeling that you were in a hospital operating room atmosphere. Because we had seen it and basically knew what was going on, I felt comfortable. . . We were wondering what it was going to be like going through the whole experience. We were in the birth room a little over 8 hours before Geoffrey was born, and then we were in there $1^1/_2$ hours after the birth.

Judy: I liked it. You didn't have to worry about being shuffled off somewhere. It's yours until you deliver.

Dennis: I enjoyed the idea of privacy, too. Our instructor/monitrice, Marcia, was there the whole time, and she was, in a sense, like part of the family. We had gotten to know her so well through the classes that she wasn't in any sense an invasion or disturbing factor at all. It was very much like home, at least from my perspective. And because the room is at the end of the hall, there wasn't a constant stream of traffic back and forth that would make you aware that you were in the middle of a very busy place. When we were walking the halls from time to time we would obviously see other people, but it was very quiet in the birth room, so you weren't aware that you were in this big hospital.

Having taken the hospital tour prior to labor helped the Reiters feel familiar with the birth room. However, mere familiarity with their environment is not what they stressed in recalling their experience. The "homey" atmosphere and privacy of the room is what they found important to them, as well as the presence of their support person, or monitrice. Social support during labor is a critical factor in improving birth experiences.[23,28]

> **Judy:** The monitrice was instrumental in getting me up to walk around. I needed to be up, but I probably wouldn't have done it on my own. I was able to hold on to both of them. She helped me off and on to the bed, encouraging me a lot. That was probably one of the biggest things. She really kept me up that way.
>
> **Dennis:** I think that part of it, too, was just her presence. She was there in the room, so, from our standpoint, if anything happened that we didn't anticipate, we would have been out of our field very quickly. The fact that we had someone there who was 10 feet away in the room was comforting, so there was no sense of worry. We never felt that she was an intruder or anything like that. Whenever I was saying something to encourage Judy she would let us have our privacy; or if I was quiet for a time, she might say something. Judy was leaning on me or her or both of us, and she held the pan for her when she felt nauseous.
>
> **Judy:** I think, too, the monitrice had seen so many births and so many different things that other people do that she could offer suggestions like, "Let's try this," or, "This might help more." That was really invaluable.

Birth experience

In the privacy of the birth room, without Judy having to move from bed to stretcher to delivery table, Geoffrey was born.

> **Dennis:** There is a sense of continuity when you are in there the whole time, and even when the doctor comes in, still it's just one more stage in an ongoing process. You're there, and you're there throughout the entire thing. But at that stage, to go through the entire labor and get right up to the end to the point where you are about to bring the baby into the world, and now you transfer to a stretcher and go across the hall and transfer to an entirely different type of atmosphere in terms of the room, I thought that would have been a really conscious break.
>
> **Judy:** Just before the head came through I was telling Denny that I didn't believe he was ever going to come out. When it actually happened and the head started to come through and then the shoulder and from there on, it was so exciting to see. Of course, we were wondering, "boy or girl?"
>
> **Dennis:** I was caught between encouraging Judy on the one hand and getting fascinated watching on the other.
>
> **Judy:** It really left you with your mouth open.
>
> **Dennis:** I really enjoyed watching this whole thing and realizing that this was

our son, although emotionally that had not hit me yet. It was a tremen-
dously positive experience.

Judy: I touched Geoffrey just as soon as he was out, and then they wrapped
him in a blanket, and I held him.

Dennis: I recall touching him before he was wrapped.

Paternal behavior at first contact

Darrell McDonald[20] videotape seven fathers immediately after the births of
their children in a homelike birth environment without intrusions. He observed
that all the fathers showed the same sequence of behavior as they contacted their
newborns for the first time. They hovered, pointed, touched the infants with their
fingertips, and then with their palms. Dennis had gingerly touched his son and
then hovered as Judy offered the baby her breast.

Dennis: Didn't the baby become quiet almost immediately as soon as you
started nursing him? You actually had him nursing at both breasts. After
about a half an hour I held him. I had made a lot of comments during the
pregnancy about how inadequate I felt I would be as a father, that I would
drop the baby and that sort of thing. That was a very, very special moment
for me. Actually I held him for about 10 minutes. I just sort of walked
around the room and bantered and talked, and he looked up at me. There
were one or two times when he made a little noise.

Judy: We were surprised that he didn't cry all that much.

Dennis: I will remember it for the rest of my life.

BRUCE AND BARBARA POSOCCO

Bruce and Barbara Posocco welcomed Jared Isaac into the world just 5 days before this interview. Labor was rapid, and the maternity unit of the hospital was busy when they arrived.

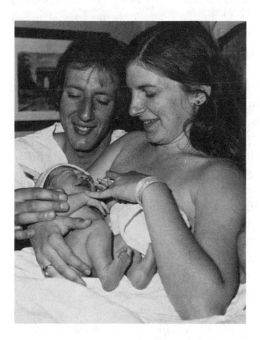

Barbara: We happened to be there on a crazy afternoon as far as deliveries, because there was lots of action going on all around.

Bruce: We didn't have a long time with those nice, short, mild contractions. We went right into those that lasted about 2 minutes. Just as one was easing up, the next one was starting. It wasn't really like a 2-minute contraction, but two really close together like a double whammie.

Barbara: I think that if everything had been a little longer, and I had had a more traditional birth, I would have made more use of the birth room, and I would have appreciated the fact that it is set up for relaxing, but by the time I got there. . . I don't even know what time I got in there really. . .

Bruce: It must have been around 2.

Barbara: The baby was born right about 3. The doctor came in a little before 2 and said that I was 8 centimeters dilated and to stop doing the breathing and to start pushing. So I was really in the birth room only about an hour. We didn't really make the use of it that is meant to be; but what I liked most, though, was staying there afterwards. At least since we were there, we didn't have to move right away afterwards.

Development of the parent-infant relationship

A quiet time alone with their baby is important to new parents as they identify their infant as a separate human being and compare what they are seeing with the fantasy baby they had lived with during the pregnancy.[16] Not having to move from a delivery room to a recovery room allows the parents uninterrupted time with their infant.

Bruce: I just couldn't describe the baby coming out. I couldn't take my eyes off him. I just had to watch. They told me that the doctor wouldn't mind if I took pictures, but I just stood there and watched. I was really amazed. I didn't touch him when he had that vernix on him. I must have touched him after about 5 or 10 minutes. I know I was on the other side of the bed.

Barbara: I thought he looked rather good from what I had expected. I had heard that some of them have even more of that sticky coating on them, or that they might have noticeable hair on their body, or even a stranger color than he was. He was blotchy and red and not like our skin. I had heard or read of all these things that our baby might look like when he was first born, so I thought he looked fairly good. I didn't think he was so ugly. I was glad that I didn't notice what the doctor was doing while he was still there. I don't know what he did besides stitches. It was a letdown kind of thing where I wasn't really concentrating on anything, so I didn't really know what he was doing. Once the doctor left, it was nice. I was glad that we could just sort of stay there and calm down a bit and come back into the real world again. It was nice to just be able to slow ourselves down a bit and take a look at the baby.

Bruce: We tried to call people. Nobody was home. I got to hold the baby, and then, after awhile, Barbara tried to put him to the breast, too. He wasn't too interested, but he had the opportunity. I'm glad that it could be that way. We don't have anything to compare it to. We didn't have a child another way, but we were very much pleased with this experience.

Barbara: I don't think we could ever have it another way.

GARY AND LINDA PANTIER

Gary and Linda Pantier were the parents of a 2½-year-old boy and a 6½-year-old girl when baby David James was born, 3 months prior to this interview. Since the births of these three children covered a span of 6½ years, interesting comparisons can be found between the Lamaze method and traditional births.

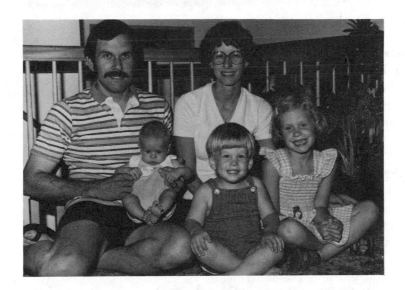

Gary: With the first baby, it was the normal-type delivery situation where the husband isn't involved at all. I wasn't even there because I spent the whole time in the waiting room. The second time we had some Lamaze training, and I could go in the labor room and in the delivery room, but the baby came so fast that time that we didn't spend much time in the labor room.

Linda: He helped me through about one contraction and that was it. I was dilated to the point where they gave me the caudal. I had to keep my hands under the drapes. Gary had to sit behind me and sit still.

Gary: We couldn't put our hands on the baby.

Linda: We couldn't even touch him or anything. Strange! For this birth I didn't have to put my feet in stirrups, and I didn't have leg drapes such as I had with the other two. The doctor just put a towel over my waist and a couple over my legs, and I just rested my legs on the bed. There wasn't really much to do, no break in my concentration at all. With the other births I was in the labor room, taken on a stretcher to the delivery room, put onto the delivery room table, draped completely; everything was covered. Even with the first baby, my arms were restrained.

Gary: While she was being wheeled down the hall, I was putting on a long gown and a cap and things like that. I went into the delivery room some time later instead of right away; I *couldn't* go in right away. When she was all ready to deliver, then they called me in, but I had to wait until then. It was much nicer this time, because before I didn't really know what was going on. The doctor was too busy, the nurses were too busy, and they didn't have any time to stop and talk to me to tell me what to expect next. I just stood in the hallway with this gown on until they finally said that I could go in, not knowing what was going on. It was much nicer this time.

Linda: I didn't like the fact that I had to keep my hands under the drape the other times. As soon as our first son was born (we had a girl first, so I was really happy to see it was a boy), I wanted to put my hand out and touch him and say, "Wow, isn't this neat!" and they were telling me, "Keep your hands under there. This is sterile in here."

Birth experience and father attachment

In a study[25] of 46 middle-income couples, the father's experience and attitude at the birth were more important than his prenatal attitude in predicting his involvement with his infant. This study was conducted from the sixth month of pregnancy to 6 months post partum with couples planning different childbirth methods, i.e, hospital birth, with and without anesthesia, and home birth. In each group, a more positive birth experience led to increased paternal attachment.

Since attachment is the foundation of caring and loving, this is very important information for personnel working with childbearing families. We believe that every effort should be made to provide a supportive and accepting birthing environment for the family.

Linda: With this birth, I can remember the doctor telling me to push just a little bit. Then once his arms were out I reached down and grabbed him and pulled him out. It was neat. The funny part was that the monitrice was telling me to look down between my legs to see the baby, but I was looking in the mirror, and all I could see was the back of the doctor's head. Finally, I got my head together and looked in the right place, and there he was! I put my hands down and pulled him up. It was really nice. It was the best part. Of course, we didn't know for a moment whether it was a boy or a girl because I just sort of pulled him up onto my stomach without really looking. Then we looked and saw it was a boy.

Gary: Linda pulled him out and a few seconds later, I guess, I had my hands on him, too. I was right there next to him. It was really neat. I hadn't been able to do that with the others. With the second one, I did carry him down the hall to the nursery, but the first one I didn't even see. I can remember thinking that it had really been great and wishing that it could have been like that with the other two.

JIM AND CAROL NORTON

Megan was 3 years old when her brother, Dylan Charles, was born at Manchester Memorial Hospital. Jim and Carol Norton had given birth in the birth room before, so the environment was not new to them.

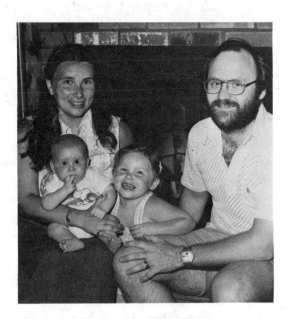

Carol: It was great to transfer to the birth room. It was like the turning point in the whole labor. You always look forward to it because it means you are really getting into it. This time, since it was the second time, it felt like going home. Plus we enjoyed not having a million other people around us. It was just the monitrice and us, and we could do our thing. Six million people didn't walk in and ask, "How're you doing?" And then at the change of shift, 6 million more people didn't come in and ask, "What's going on and how're you doing?" That was really nice. The nurses were real nice people—I don't mean anthing against them. It was just the constant hassle of being bothered all the time by a variety of people and not knowing if they were really worrying about me. I sat there wondering where the nurse was, did she forget about me, things like that, before we transferred to the birth room with our own monitrice.

Carol's dislike of having to relate to numerous people and their messages while laboring is a common complaint of childbearing women today. Laboring women are increasingly objecting to being treated as if they are ill, and in the process being scrutinized by numerous hospital staff members.

Dylan was born after about 7 hours of labor.

Carol: Wow! It was easier to pay attention this time because I knew what to expect and what to look for. Just to see that little head coming out and watching the doctor suctioning him, these are things that you always think of as happening to someone else and not actually happening to you. Then he slippy-slides the little kid right out. I touched him immediately after he was born. His head had so much vernix on it. That's the first thing I started touching—rubbing the vernix on his scalp.

Jim: It was just a tremendous surge. It's kind of indescribable. It's an emotion that I've never felt before other than with Megan's birth. I guess it's mixed relief that it's happened, and Carol is all right, and there's what we've been working on all these months. It's over, and it's just starting. It's really indescribable. Dylan was on her stomach and chest, and initially I was just able to say "hello" and rub his back a little bit. I held him later on.

Carol: The baby was wide awake, eyes open. I can't remember either baby crying, not even right after they were born. I just remember them with their eyes wide open, just looking and staring with that cute baby stare. Touching him, rubbing that vernix in, feeling that unique newness of him, looking at that awful color of him, knowing that his head will get back into shape, thinking, just looking at all the different parts, you know, just looking at what you've been working on for 9 months. Just making sure that they are all there. I nursed both babies for a short while. Both times I was still very shaky, so it wasn't very easy for me.

Jim: I really don't think the bonding time is long enough. It's easy for me to say that I'd like to have the newborn with the family right away and all the time, knowing that Carol needs her rest and all. But I still don't think it was long enough. I'd be much happier if the babies were never in the nursery. I just won't like the nursery environment. I don't even much care to go down and see all the babies just lying there, row by row.

Bonding

Jim expressed a need for more bonding time beyond the hour they all shared as a family. His initial contact with Dylan had been to say hello and rub his back a little bit. It wasn't until later that he held his son, and then he didn't want to let him go. What he was experiencing was an early affectional bond formation, a period of assessment for both father and son as they began attaching to one another.

Attachment, as defined by Klaus and Kennell,[16] is " a unique relationship between two people that is specific and endures through time." Attachment is the very foundation of caring and loving, the original mother-infant, father-infant bond that continues through a lifetime.

Klaus and Kennell[16] have published studies that question whether the damaging relationship that occurs in animals when mother and offspring are separated also occurs in humans. "Cows and ewes, for instance, that are separated from their young ones for 1 or 2 hours after birth are found to neglect and abuse their off-spring." The authors say that "eight out of nine studies conducted in other countries on humans show that mothers and newborns will have considerably closer relationship if allowed to have more contact immediately following birth than traditional hospital practices allow. The time immediately after birth in humans as in animals may be an important 'bonding' or 'attachment' period for mother and baby." Klaus and Kennell, who together directed a mother-infant research unit at Case Western Reserve University, Cleveland, studied two groups of first-time mothers for 2 years after they had given birth. The 14 mothers in one group had the traditional glimpse of their baby after birth, a brief contact between 6 and 12 hours later, and visits of 20 to 30 minutes every hour for bottle feeding. The 14 mothers in the experiemental group had 16 additional hours of contact, including 1 hour of contact with their nude baby under a heat panel within the first 3 hours of birth. The studies concluded that the mothers who had extended contact developed considerably more emotional, mental, and physical ties with their children than did the control group mothers. Klaus' research team checked the mothers 1 month, 1 year, and 2 years after the time of birth. The experimental group mothers, he said, were more attentive to their babies, spoke to them more, asked twice as many questions, and made half as many demands as the control group women. He concludes that the initial 45-minute visit with the baby after birth appears to be an important rendezvous time for mother and child.

Peter de Chateau[8] reviewed numerous studies on the importance of the neonatal period for development of mother-infant attachment. In this review, he maintains that what happens in the period immediately following birth is very important in the development of mother-infant-father relationships. The importance of early maternal closeness, feeding, and infant stimulation appeared consistently in the studies reviewed. Father-infant interactions in the period after birth may be just as important for the infant when evaluating affectional bond formation.

In 1974 Greenberg[10] stated that the period within the first 3 days after birth is the interval in which fathers begin developing a bond with their newborn. In this research, the term "engrossment" was coined to describe the characteristics of this bond, observable in clinic interviews. These characteristics include a feeling of preoccupation, absorption, and interest in the newborn along with a desire to look at, hold, and touch him. According to Greenberg, "the early contact by the father with the newborn seems to be significant in releasing engrossment."

Sibling participation

In addition to feeling the need for a longer bonding time, Jim expressed a desire to share more of this experience with their older child. With people now actively preparing for birth, sibling involvement in the entire process is a phenomenon that is growing. Classes in preparation for birth are being offered for siblings, and some hospitals and birth centers are including siblings at births. Research is needed in this area before sibling participation in births can be encouraged on a universal scale.[2] However, to reduce sibling rivalry and maternal-child separation anxiety, it is important to include siblings in the hospital experience as much as possible.

Jim: I think there should be some effort made to include the whole family a little bit more. The sibling visitation that one time was all right, but I was kind of disappointed. Megan was real excited about getting to see her mom and to go down to see the baby, but I guess I would have rather have had all that happen at home and not spent the time in the hospital to begin with. I guess it would have been best for us if Carol had been able to stay in the hospital and recuperate, and the baby could have come home with us. The family could have gotten off on a start together. You recognize that the rest and relaxation is needed, but the hospital is not the place for the baby to be in. There is no family togetherness in the hospital. The sibling visitation just does not go far enough.

Carol: I don't know if you'd want to expose her to the whole birthing experience.

Jim: No, we probably wouldn't want to do that. She *has* seen all the pictures.

Carol: She might have been ready for it. It might have given her some thoughts about her own birth, too. You never can tell.

Jim: Mostly it just gave her thoughts of being pregnant.

Carol: One day I was running down the street, and I said that I just couldn't run any more, and she sat down and said, "Mom, I'm so tired of being pregnant!"

DICK AND JULIE MULLER

Twenty-four hours after Julie's membranes had ruptured, Dick and Julie Muller arrived at the hospital for an induction. Although they had seen pictures of the birth room, they had not toured the hospital.

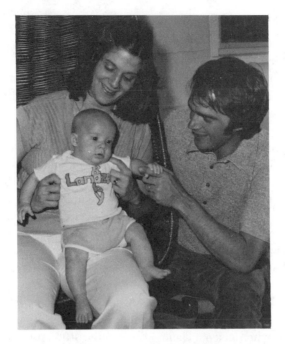

Dick: It was quite a contrast as we went by the delivery rooms with their tile floors and sterile environment.

Julie: The birth room had pictures and really looked inviting. The other delivery rooms looked like they'd be scary.

Dick: Our room was small enough to be cozy.

Julie: I felt comfortable in there and liked the privacy. I wouldn't have liked to have someone on the other side of the curtain going through labor and hearing everything. This way we could talk privately and joke around and say whatever we wanted to. Dick ate his lunch out in the hall; it was after I had the paracervical block, and I got up and went out with him. I sat in the rocking chair, and they plugged in the monitor out there. The sun was streaming in the French windows, and I just couldn't believe that *we* were so relaxed, just sitting there in the sun and looking forward to the birth.

Dick: The only really rough time was just before Julie was fully dilated. She was working really hard then, and went in and out of the bathroom, and it was really hot.

Julie: That's another thing. In the regular labor room, the bathroom was so narrow that I wouldn't have been able to use it at all because of the monitor and the IVAC. That was the coolest place, so I spent quite a bit of time in there while I was in labor.

Ambulation in labor

In a study[9] of 68 women in spontaneous labor, half labored in a recumbent position whereas half labored while ambulatory. The results showed that the ambulatory women had a shorter labor than those in bed. Also, the ambulatory women needed less analgesia and less oxytocic augmentation than the recumbent women.

Dr. Roberto Caldeyro-Barcia[14] of Montevideo, Uruguay, President of the International Federation of Gynecologists and Obstetricians and Director of the Latin American Center for Perinatology and Human Development of the World Health Organization, feels, on the basis of extensive clinical research, that labor and delivery are "natural physiological processes, which should proceed normally and with very little intervention from those who are taking care of the mother and the neonate if everything is normal, which is the truth in 80% to 85% of cases." Caldeyro-Barcia's[7] study on the influence of maternal position during the second stage of labor indicated that duration of the second stage could be significantly reduced by the upright position of the woman.

Recent research[21] indicates that when women stand in first-stage labor, they experience more efficient uterine contractions and less discomfort than women lying in bed. Also, when given a choice, the women studied preferred the standing position.

Julie believes that being able to move about during labor was a definite asset for her. To have their own "space" and to be able to come and go in that space served to hasten the labor for Julie and Dick.

Julie: When I was ready to give birth I was cleaned, and then the doctor came in and made his sterile field. The table was changed. At first it was like a bed. Then the leg supports came up from somewhere, I guess, I don't know from where. I really wasn't aware of what was going on; I can hardly remember. I did feel like I was going to fall for a minute, because the lower part of the bed wasn't there, but everyone reassured me that my legs were supported and that I was OK, so then I felt more secure. Otherwise, I don't really remember that part at all.

Dick: The contractions were coming so quick, I can't see how she could have moved at that point.

Julie: It was exciting. I remember the monitrice telling me to keep my eyes open. Then we heard him gurgle when he was still inside. I'll just always remember that sound. It was just so exciting to look down and see his little face. Even during labor, I don't think I attached any kind of physical structure to the baby, it was just something that had been there. When I heard him gurgle, ooh, I can still remember the chills that I got from hearing it.

Dick: I remember looking down when his head first came out. His head was kind of elongated and blue. The doctor immediately suctioned out his mouth and nose and worked at getting the shoulders out. Before he even got him out he was already pink.

Julie: We have pictures of him halfway out. Then the doctor got him the rest of the way out and just held him up to me, and I got to hold him right away. He was probably a minute old.

Dick: The cord was still attached. He placed the baby right on her stomach. I guess I touched him, too. Yes, I did; I touched his arm. He was very clean. We had seen pictures of babies with lots of that cheesy stuff on them, but aside from a little blood he was very clean. He was wet looking. He looked mad. He started to fuss, and then she fed him right away, and he calmed down and kept one eye open.

Julie: That was another thing that the monitrice did. I had never breastfed a baby before. I needed help with that. He started eating right away, and his little eyes opened, and he looked around.

Breastfeeding

Julie's experience with breastfeeding is not an isolated one, since for human mothers breastfeeding is not an instinctive act. Women learning to breastfeed need instruction and support.[11] With the baby awake, alert, and in a first reactive phase immeditely after birth, nurses have an excellent opportunity to support the family new to breastfeeding. Just as Julie needed help, so do many women.

Maternal medication

For women to be successful with breastfeeding, it is important that the baby be alert and not depressed by barbiturates given to the mother in labor. Numerous studies have demonstrated transient effects on the behavior of neonates born to medicated mothers. In one study of babies of 41 multiparous mothers who had nursed a previous baby, Brazelton[6] reported a 24- to 48-hour time lag in the baby's ability to adapt to breastfeeding. A study by Kron and associates[18] found that routine maternal medication in labor depressed newborn sucking behavior significantly for 4 days after delivery. Studies by Scanlon and associates,[27] and by Brackbill and associates,[4] demonstrated that maternal medication may affect neonatal neurologic functioning. There have been many more studies demonstrating the effect of medication on infants since Brazelton's[5] article on the "Effect of Prenatal

Drugs on the Behavior of the Neonate" back in 1970, and yet, little has been done to change the routine medication of laboring mothers with tranquilizers and barbiturates.

That Lamaze preparation for labor and delivery has the potential to reduce or eliminate a laboring woman's use of narcotics is demonstrated in a controlled study by Scott and Rose.[28] They compared the labor and delivery characteristics of 129 nulliparous women who had Lamaze preparation with an equal number of matched control subjects who had not had Lamaze preparation. The prepared women required significantly fewer narcotics during labor, had fewer forceps deliveries, and received conduction anesthesia less often.

A study by Huttel and colleagues,[13] comparing 31 Lamaze-prepared nulliparas with 41 control patients, also showed that the prepared women, who had their husbands with them, required significantly less medication than the control group.

STEVE AND PAM CARTER

Steve and Pam Carter recalled the birth of their first son, David Miles, 4 months after his birth.

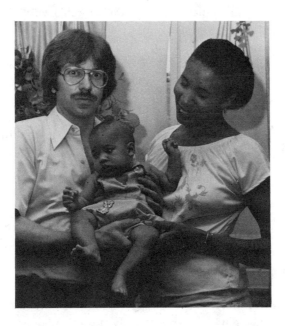

Steve: The first thing that happened after we arrived at the hospital was a nurse came in and wanted to give Pam a shot. They put her in bed, and the lady came in and said, "I'm going to give you a shot for your pain." The nurse wanted me to leave, but I didn't want to because I was afraid that she would talk Pam into taking the shot. I was determined to go through the whole process with her, and I wasn't going to get gypped by anyone talking me into leaving on whatever excuse it was: that I needed sleep, or whatever.

Pam: I was really getting uncomfortable, and that's when the nurse said to Steve that he could go lie down in some room somewhere and to me that she could give me a shot or a pill.

Steve: I asked her what was in it. I had to ask her twice before she told me that it was Demerol. So I said no, *we* didn't want that. I told her *we* were going to use our breathing.

Pam: At that point, I was going to say yes to the shot.

Steve: That's why I insisted on staying with her, because we had agreed during the pregnancy that we would go for a paracervical block if she needed something. Since I was more confident that the breathing would work than Pam was, I was determined to try.

Role of nursing

A laboring woman complaining of pain and showing obvious signs of pain can create anxiety for the nurse as well as for herself and her family. As the nurse assesses the woman's pain, quick intervention for relief with medication is often suggested. However, for Steve and Pam, this nurse failed to follow through her assessment. Steve explained persistently that they had attended prenatal classes and wanted an unmedicated delivery. The nurse is responsible for helping the family obtain the safest and most positive childbirth experience; however, insisting on medication was not compatible with the Carters' plans for their labor and birth, especially Steve's.

Although it was several hours before a monitrice arrived and the Carters moved with her to the birth room, with Steve's support and constant attendance Pam was able to labor without medication.

Pam: After the monitrice came and we went down to the birth room, I felt much more relaxed. I felt I had privacy and could go into labor in peace and had nothing to worry about.

Steve: I was tired, We had just come through the 2-hour period of fighting off the nurses. I was more relaxed by that time because the monitrice was on my side. I knew I could slip away to have some food without having somebody give Pam a pill. At that point I was ready to go all the way down the line. *We* were trained very well. *We* knew what we were doing. *We* had practiced every night, so *we* were ready. I was confident that it would work. Although Pam was less confident that I was, I was confident that *we* were going to do it. *We* were just going to do it and that was it! I was actively involved the whole time because I wanted to be and didn't want to miss this one chance that I probably was going to have.

Concept of control

Control of their experience was very important for this couple. According to Morris,[22] birth preparation classes "enable women to approach labor with confidence and bring it under their own control." Although control means different things to different people, the nurse's challenge is to help each childbearing family have a sense of control. Willmuth[35] reviewed the retrospective evaluations of 145 women in a prepared childbirth program and found that their perception of maintaining control was closely associated with satisfaction. In this study, maintaining control meant many things, ranging from control of pain perception, to control over one's emotions and actions, to control in interpersonal relationships with staff.

According to Rubin,[26] loss of control in any form may result in loss of self-esteem and bring on a feeling of shame and humiliation. By insisting on giving medication for pain, despite Steve's refusal, the nurse described here was seen by the Carters as a threat to their control and ultimately to their self-esteem.

With the support of their monitrice, the Carters were able to regain control over their experience. That this control contributed to their satisfaction is obvious as they relate the birth.

Pam: At the time of the birth, I remember having my eyes closed. I remember Steve telling me first to push; then he said, "I can see the head." Then I would push again and he'd see more head. My eyes were closed and I remember feeling that I just couldn't do it. That was just as the head was coming out. Then the monitrice said, "Open your eyes, open your eyes." So I opened my eyes and looked in the mirror. I gave a real hard push. I could feel the doctor pushing down on my perineum. Then the head came out, and it felt like a real big relief. I just couldn't believe it. I saw the baby's face as the doctor aspirated his mouth and nose. Seconds later, the whole body came out. The doctor gave him right to me. That I thought was unusual, because I was waiting for them to wipe David up and everything, and I don't know if I had my arms out or what I did. I was in complete awe, looking at the baby's face and how small he was. I didn't bother to look to see what sex it was, because at that point it was just a baby. The baby was ours, mine, and in my arms, and I couldn't believe that I did it. I couldn't believe that I'd done the whole job. I remember Steven whispering in my ear and telling me, "It's a boy." And then I just called him "David." It was like an awesome experience. Unbelievable! I never thought in my life that I could have a baby like that. I had thought that I would always be put to sleep. Us girls, when we were younger, talking about it, I would say, "If I have a baby, they'll put me to sleep, knock me out for sure." This was unbelievable. It was beautiful. Steve said he wished he had a recording of it, because I went from instant doubt to instant awe.

Steve: What I remember was seeing more and more of the hair every time she pushed, and a lot more of his head. I remember the doctor telling her to stop pushing at one point, so the head wouldn't pop out. I told her to blow to stop her pushing, which she did as soon as I did it, she copied me. That made me feel good. I was still in there, being important. Then the head came out, and David made noises right away, which made me feel great, because I knew he was alive. The first thing I remember was that he started gurgling. I felt really good. OK, he's breathing and he's fine. Only his head was out. His chest wasn't out yet. His shoulders didn't clear yet. He was making little noises. I was really happy. Then the shoulders came out. The rest of him just slid right out. I saw it was a boy. I had to look. The doctor cut the cord really quick and put him on Pam's stomach. He worked very fast and very gently, which was really good compared to the pictures we'd seen where doctors slapped babies to wake them up. That's probably why I was so happy that he was gurgling when his head came out, because I knew nobody would have to hit him. He didn't cry; he was gurgling, but he never had to cry. As soon as I saw he was a boy, I said to Pam, "He's a boy." Within the space of about 5 or 6 seconds she went from saying, "I can't do it, I can't do it," to "David, David." That was almost tearful. I wish I'd had a tape recording of the last 3 or 4 minutes. Pam held him. She was just looking at him. He had his little, long fingers in front of his face, so you couldn't see him. He had his eyes open, though. He seemed to be trying to look, which was very exciting. He was a red, little scrawny thing. Then I remember the doctor reminding us that the placenta had to come. We knew that. At that point we didn't care, at least I didn't care.

Pam: I remember wanting to cry all the time, but I didn't. I remember holding him. Then I thought he was getting cold, so I asked the nurse to take him and wrap him up. She did, and she brought him back to me. At that time I don't know if she put the drops in his eyes. I think she did. Everything seemed so fast. The hour went by fast. Then Steve held the baby for a good while and talked to him.

Steve: I held him for a good 20 to 30 minutes. The only thing I was worried about was that it was too cold in the room for him. I really enjoyed holding him and seeing his little fingers in front of his face. I wasn't afraid. It was really nice. I was proud, and I was proud to be there. I was proud that *We* had done it, and that *we* had done it together. The bonding wasn't just between me and the baby, it was between me and Pam and the baby. It was like *we* had done something special together, which we will never forget. I'll never forget it, and I know Pam will never forget it.

Pam: Believe it or not, we still talk about it, and every time we both feel like we want to cry again. That's how beautiful it was. I remember we kept talking about it during the first few weeks. We just kept reminding each other about it. We just get a big lump in our throats, and we feel like crying.

Steve: Sometimes that helps us through the bad times, when he cries all night.

RUSS AND BETSY TONKIN

When Betsy and Russ Tonkin shared the birth of Tara 4 months ago, they carried with them the memories of Heather's birth 2½ years previously. Since Heather had been born in a traditional hospital setting, they could compare the two experiences.

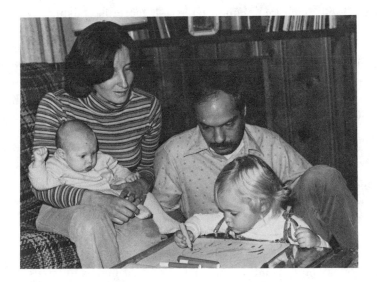

Both Betsy and Russ had seen the Lamaze room before labor actually began, so their labor and birth environment was not a surprise. Betsy recalled her first impression of the room:

Betsy: Blue! My first impression was blue! When I walked into the room, I first noticed the color, the walls, the curtains, the pictures. It was very nice, more like walking into a room rather than the usual sterile environment that you would ordinarily connect with the hospital. It was a much softer feeling.

Russ: It was a much warmer feeling than the labor room that Betsy was in when we had Heather. That one was all white with a hospital bed, and it was all sterile looking. This one was more like a room. The rocker was there. There were pictures on the wall. Touches like that made it much nicer.

Betsy: We were actually in the Lamaze room about 2 hours before Tara was born. I was up and about. I started out in the rocking chair and thought that was just glorious! The rocking chair was lovely, and I remember thinking at that time how nice it is to have a rocking chair because it does make it very homey, very comfortable, very natural, very unlike the situation where Heather was born. For that labor I went into the labor room and was immediately put into bed, and that's where I stayed for the duration of labor. When I was thinking about it afterwards, I thought that in a conventional labor room everything is geared to, well, sickness. And pregnancy, labor, and delivery is not a sickness. The first labor room made me more introverted. I can remember lying in bed with contractions and just thinking about the next contraction and the next. Whereas rocking in the rocking chair, I felt much more comfortable, felt more like talking, looking around. There were other things in the room and other people in the room: the monitrice and Russ. It was much happier, much calmer, much more peaceful than the labor room where I labored with Heather. The first time all I wanted to do was curl up and let the contractions come over me and take over. I felt introverted. The Lamaze room made me feel much more like throwing my thoughts outward. . . more natural. I thought it was wonderful. I was rocking and we were chatting; once I got up and went to the bathroom—all by myself! Before I could never do that. Once you were in bed with the monitor attached, that's where you stayed. And I had a long, 10-hour labor!

Birth environment

Betsy describes very clearly the effect of the environment on a laboring woman when she talks about the first labor room making her feel more introverted. As labor progresses, women tend to lose control of their bodies to forces within them. A controlling, sterile, unfamiliar, and unnatural environment can compound this sense of loss of control.[12]

Through the work of B. F. Skinner[30-32] and numerous behavioral psychologists, we have been made aware of the effect of the environment on human behavior. These scientists have shown us that it is possible to design an environment in which one can direct control of an individual. Change the environment and you change the behavior.

There are also a wealth of studies demonstrating that specific environments in hospitals definitely affect people's recovery.[1,15,24] Color, the presence of monitors and other technical equipment, and even the size of the hospital room are very important. In a hospital in the Washington, D.C., area, it was found that certain patients deteriorated rapidly when being cared for in a very small room.[15] A comparison[36] of 77 patients' feelings in single-care and two-bed rooms showed that 64% of those in single rooms experienced sensory disturbances. However, only 34% of those people in two-bed rooms experienced sensory disturbances during their hospitalization. The presence of another person in the room was very important in reducing signs of sensory deprivation.

Understanding the concept of sensory alteration may be crucial to understanding how birth room environments influence labor. Sensory alteration encompasses sensory deprivation and sensory overload.[1] Most researchers describe sensory deprivation as decreases in the amount or intensity of stimulation. Coexistent with sensory deprivation can be perceptual deprivation, which refers to reduction in the meaningfulness of the stimulation. Too little stimulation can be as disruptive as too much stimulation, or sensory overload. Also, the amount of stimulation, level of stimulus variation, and meaning of the stimulation are important.[29]

Since most laboring people are young and well, they often have never been hospitalized before their labor experience. A standard hospital labor room, stripped of any familiar amenities such as pictures, drapes, and homelike furniture, provides an immediate decrease in the sensory input to which they are accustomed. If they are then confined without family or friends to this one small, unfamiliar, windowless room, the couple is further deprived of familiar and meaningful stimuli. Add to their altered sensory and perceptual fields hospital routines, technical language, and electronic equipment and the result can be the cognitive and emotional deterioration of sensory alteration—or as Betsy described it, "a feeling of introversion."

Introducing people to the labor and birth environment before delivery day can help to reduce the strangeness of that environment for them. But even more important is providing meaningful sensory input in that environment, which is what the birth room does.

In comparing their first birth experience with Tara's birth, the Tonkins present a beautiful example of active participation. As they relate this experience, notice how the physician and nurses encouraged them to accept responsibility for their infant's birth. As a result, Betsy was not delivered; she gave birth.

Betsy: The doctor was very helpful. I can remember him giving me very specific instructions, always telling me what he was going to do before he did it: "I'm going to iron out the perineum now. Watch your progress in the mirror. Open your eyes." The monitrice also said, "Let your body tell you what to do." I remember that. The doctor said, "Here's the head. Look in the mirror. Stop pushing and blow when I tell you." Always sort of one step ahead, so we always knew what to expect and what I was going to feel next.

One of the things that surprised me was that by my lifting her out, she was facing toward me and the doctor said, "Well, what do you have, a boy or a girl?" And I remember thinking, "Oh, my gosh, what a switch, the obstetrician asking the mother the sex of the baby. Usually it's the other way around." This time I got to tell him. It was a very nice tone of things. I wanted to reach down after the head was out and pull my baby out the rest of the way, which the doctor and monitrice helped me to do. I was a little unsure as to just when was the right time to reach down, but the monitrice guided my hands, and I reached under Tara's hands and I remember thinking, "What do I do now?" and just then the doctor said, "Now, lift and push." Then it all made sense to me. So I pushed once and lifted her out and put her right up onto my chest. That was a beautiful feeling.

I remember that with the first delivery, I did the majority of pushing in the labor room, and then when it was time to go to the delivery room, I can remember being wheeled out and down the hall. Russ was gone. He had to go somewhere else to get his cap and mask and wash his hands and put his shoe coverings on. Then I had to move from the stretcher to the delivery table, and there was this big hump that they try to push down, but it still was in the way. And of course during all of this I was still having contractions and wanting to push, and they were saying, "Don't push!" It was very hard trying to move over. So there were a lot of distractions: the move to the stretcher, the ride down the hall, everything is changing as you go by, then the difficult move at an inopportune time. Russ wasn't there, and I was having contractions and wanting to push. Of course there was the IV bottle that had to be transferred, and we had to be careful of the IV tubing, and my legs were put in the stirrups, strapped in, and covered. And then the drapes were put on. So there was a lot they had to do to get me ready the first time. I must have had at least three or four contractions during that time. Then too, the delivery room is a whole different environment. It was cold! And very, very bright. This time in the birth room, the lights were dimmed and the shades were pulled down.

Russ: This time I was really fascinated watching what was going on. I was a lot closer to the birth. The first time I was up by her head, actually behind Betsy so I couldn't see as much.

Betsy: The thing I wanted most of all from this delivery was to be able to touch the baby. I felt I was greatly deprived of this the first time around. This was one of the things that enthralled me this time, to be able to actually touch the baby right at time of delivery and to be able to hold her as close as possible. That touching made all the difference in the world to me. Our monitrice handed Russ a towel and told him to pat and rub the baby dry.

Russ: Yes, I touched her probably 30 seconds after she was born.

Betsy: Russ dried her off. The doctor was in no hurry to cut the cord. Eventually he did. The monitrice put the little stockinette cap on her and checked her position to facilitate drainage. She was a little mucusy, so she positioned her with her head down, but she wasn't taken from me.

It's pretty hard to put it into words. The touching was so important. The first time I could only put my hand up over the bassinet. It was actually a fingertip touching. That was all. With Tara I could not only touch, but hold close. I can remember feeling that she was warm, she was wet, she was slippery; that feeling of her warm, wet body on my body transcends every-thing. I just can't explain it. I can remember my arms enfolding her—not a touch as much as my arms went all the way around her. All I could say was, "You're beautiful. I can't believe this." Things like that. It was too wonderful. That's what I was feeling right afterward. Then of course, coming down a little bit. The feeling of having the intensity of labor and delivery behind and just looking at this baby and knowing that she was ours, knowing that we really took a part in bringing her into the world. For both of us, it was just marvelous. I'd do it again and again.

JIM AND PAT SULLIVAN

Jim and Pat Sullivan experienced a long, hard labor when Timothy was born. Recalling their experience 3 months later, the importance of the labor team was obvious.

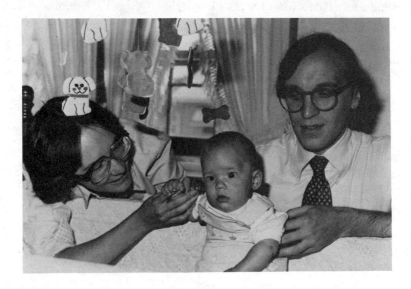

Jim: I stayed with her the whole time. I'll never forget it. Here it was 3 A.M., and after they got through with the preliminary paperwork we went upstairs. They asked me if I wanted to go down to the fathers' waiting room, and I said, "No." They said that all they were going to do was to prep Pat and give her an enema, I think. And I said, "So?" And they asked if I really wanted to stay with her for all of that, and I said that I didn't see why not. We had started this together; we'll keep going together. The nurse said that that would be fine; it didn't make any difference to her. Pat was sort of insistent that I stay with her, too.

Pat: During labor we walked down to the nursery several times and walked all over the area. That helped! Then in the Lamaze room, if it hadn't been for Jim and the monitrice rubbing my back 99% of the time with their hands, I don't know how I would have done what I did. Having that much support really helped, because there was really nothing that I could have done for my own back. Another thing that the monitrice suggested was pushing on my side. I don't know if I would ever have thought of doing that myself had I been there by myself or just with my husband. And that side-pushing really helped.

Jim: I was chief surgeon! [Laughter] I am a frustrated doctor! In my last year of college, I realized that I should have gone to med school, but not being that proficient in math I realized that I probably couldn't do it. So this was my first experience in the "operating arena!" [Laughter] No, seriously, my function there, I think the role I played, was an important one. I wasn't just an adjunct. I was an important part of this whole thing. Emotionally I think, for Pat, it was good to have me there. This whole thing was sort of a joint effort, as it is probably best put. It only seemed natural that I should be there and not abandon her to the uncertainties of birth. . . and there are uncertainties.

I ran through everything I learned in our Lamaze classes from the wet washcloth—and when that warmed up, I fanned it to cool it—and all these other things. I think we used just about everything. The only thing that we didn't use was the socks. She never put on the socks that I bought her for Christmas: those big, beautiful, red socks with black snowflakes. But most important, I was there. I was part of it. I was emotionally and physically involved in the whole process. I was not at all uncomfortable; I felt really needed.

Pat: Our monitrice gave any support and encouragement that was needed at any time. Even though we had been extremely well-prepared in our class, there were still some things that we forgot or didn't anticipate. She offered suggestions so that every part of my body was in the right place to give me the least amount of pain or trouble. She gave me constant coaching, and I think that had I been alone or in a situation where a nurse ran in maybe every 10 minutes, I might have gotten very frustrated. And although I wouldn't say that I might have panicked, I would have had a lot more difficulty. Also, she was able to give extra support on the back where two hands did not do the job. That was a great big help.

Jim: I think her role was almost that of a coach. We were the players and she made suggestions. It's like when you're in a game: the players have to carry out the game plan, the actions. The coach can make suggestions after having been there or having experienced these things at least one time before, and is detached from the action in some respects and has an overview that was important.

Pat: I always had the feeling that she didn't want to interfere with anything if we just wanted to do something on our own, but she was always there if we needed the help, or suggestions, or support. This was nice because it was *our* experience, and we wanted to direct it as much as possible. But certainly the help was something that, unless you've been there, you don't really appreciate how important this person is to you. In looking back on it, I'm more and more convinced that the monitrice is the way to go.

Labor team

The importance of a labor-support team cannot be overemphasized. Frequently, nursing staffs tend to let a Lamaze couple alone to "do their own thing," feeling that they are well-prepared and in control. The term "coach" is often used to designate or describe a laboring woman's support person. Notice that Jim and Pat felt that the monitrice was their coach. It was their first experience "playing the game together," and their experienced monitrice was directing or coaching. Expecting an inexperienced, expectant father to be "coach" may be unrealistic and totally ignore his needs in the birth experience.

When speaking about the actual birth, it became obvious what effect the team can have on a father's experience. Since Jim and Pat were being supported by other team members, Jim was free to experience the birth to its fullest—relieved of "coaching" duties.

Jim: It got to the point where we knew the birth was imminent, from my perspective anyway. I had my camera there, and I knew I should be taking pictures, but I thought that if I looked away I might miss something. I felt that this was the first time that I was ever involved in anything like this, and I really didn't want to look through anything but my own eyes and sort of record it through my own memory. I was just totally caught up in the whole process. When the episiotomy was done—we had all heard what the episiotomy was—I can't say that I was shocked by it, but I was astounded as to how it was done. I'm not sure what I expected. I guess I expected a little snip, but the doctor did a real good cut with a pair of scissors twice. I thought to myself, "Oh, my goodness." When the forceps were inserted, then it was just incredible. It was the culmination of 30-plus hours of anxious anticipation and of emotional preparation. Then to see him being born! There was a point where his head and shoulders were out, and he was making the turn, and I looked down and could see him taking his first breath. I don't know how much he was actually taking in at that time, but his mouth was moving. It was kind of a strange experience. The rest of the birth was very easy, after the head and shoulders. And at one point before the doctor had inserted the forceps, he kind of shook his head. I'm sure it was just an unconscious gesture, but I saw it and thought something was wrong. After that he didn't seem concerned, but after a bit when he realized that it was a compound presentation, he seemed relieved. He said, "Oh, here's the problem, he's got his hand up by his head!" That was the only thing that was just a little unusual. After he was born, our first concern was not whether he was a boy or girl, because at the point it really didn't matter. As a matter of fact, the doctor asked if we didn't want to look and see what we had.

Pat: That became very unimportant at the time.

Jim: Right, the gender was unimportant at the time: just the fact that he was healthy and had all his hands and toes, and they seemed to be all there. Then it was, by the way, we have a boy! That was great too.

Pat: I was very interested in seeing Jim's reaction, too, not just for myself. I was so anxious to see my husband experiencing this. I could feel things but I was interested in his emotions, too.

Jim: It was truly the most emotional experience that I've ever been through. When he was born, and he was out, and we knew it was a boy, then there is sort of a lag time. It doesn't set in immediately. Then I began to realize that this is a real person; this is a little living being, and he's mine. It's just incredible! It's an amazing experience.

ERIC AND SANDY OZOLS

When remembering the birth of Tara 7 months earlier, Sandy illustrates how an awake and aware, positive birth experience can influence mothering.

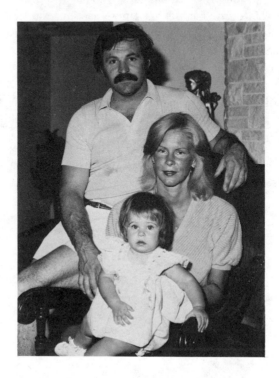

Sandy: I was working so hard. I'm glad that Eric was there because he told me to look at the important part, or I would have missed the whole thing. He said, "Look, the baby's head." It happened so fast! I thought that it would come in stages, you know, first the head would be out, then 5 or 10 minutes later the shoulders would come, but it just happened so easy at that point.

Eric: Once the head was out, the rest of the body just slipped out.

Sandy: I'll never forget that feeling, being awake. No matter how much pain you have to go through, I would do it over and over. I wrote it down in my baby book just as soon as I came home from the hospital because I was afraid that I would forget the words that I felt, the feeling that came over me when the doctor helped her out and put her on my stomach. I was in tears.

Eric: I got a picture of that. We can actually see where she is crying.

Sandy: You could just see it on my face. It just brings tears to my eyes when I talk about it. It was such an emotional feeling when the doctor brought her up and placed her here. She was really screaming and crying, but it was just so emotional. I really have no words to describe it, just that instinct that I was a mother took right over me. I was really a mother! And from that day I've been a marshmallow! The feelings that I got were really overwhelming. . . and to miss that, no matter how much pain I had to go through, it's worth it to see it, to be right there, instead of being knocked out.

Mothering

Sandy describes the instinct that took over at Tara's birth and of knowing she was "really a mother." The importance of being alert and awake, and of immediate touching in the mother-infant relationship cannot be overemphasized. In Sandy's instance, this initial bonding experience carried over to provide a positive milieu for breastfeeding.

Sandy: I was the one that wasn't going to breastfeed. I just had a thing about it. My mother said that I had to breastfeed. Everybody told me that I had to, I just *had* to. Well, I felt I didn't have to if I didn't want to. I asked Eric what he thought. He suggested that I at least try it, so I decided that I would. I bought only one maternity bra, because I didn't think that I was going to last. Well as soon as they brought that little baby into my room— well, I tried to breastfeed her right in the Lamaze room, but she wouldn't take it—but when they brought her into my room for that first feeding, that little face, that little nose, she was so cute that I loved it. Now I just talk about it to everyone: "You have to breastfeed!" Now I'm the same way. It's a really nice, close experience. I wouldn't do it any other way. I'd never go with the bottle.

That the Ozols' positive birth experience influenced their parenting is apparent when they talk of themselves as man, woman, wife, and husband.

Sandy: I remember when we were single and talking to married couples who were always talking about their children coming first. I would say, "No, your husband should always come first. He's your mate. After the children are married you still have him."

Eric: We just couldn't conceive of children coming first. But now when Tara gives us a big smile, it's all over.

Sandy: I get a feeling: "motherhood." I don't know if Eric feels it as much as I do. But right from the beginning, right there in the hospital, I was a different person. It just took right over, this feeling, this instinct, this motherhood instinct. I don't neglect Eric. I'd read a lot of books explaining how the husband feels left out after a baby is born. So I told him that I had to spend a lot of time with the baby now because I'm nursing, and can't spend as much time with him. He said that he understood. We just talked and more or less told each other how it was going to be. Even now Tara is still nursing, and she does require quite a bit of time. We know that later on it will be different.

Published evaluative studies[3] of psychoprophylaxis in childbirth have been criticized for not using appropriate control groups. The interviews presented so far in this chapter are simply representative of couples who chose to attend childbirth classes and use a monitrice in the Lamaze room at Manchester Memorial Hospital. Although they do not represent the use of experimental methodology, we feel that these interviews present evidence that a positive birth has the power to influence and to change peoples' lives for the better. The couples who shared their birth experiences with the interviewer talked of the importance of a "homey" atmosphere and a support person in reducing their anxiety during labor. They spoke of the value that having some control over their environment had to their feelings of self-esteem. The benefit of father participation in the birth to the quality of the experience itself, as well as to father-attachment, was emphasized. That childbirth education can reduce fear and anxiety was perhaps best illustrated by the feeling in labor of "controlled excitement" that one couple described. Each couple related the significance their bonding time alone as a family for an hour after birth had for self-concepts of mothering and fathering.

In the following pages are interviews with a few couples who did not choose the monitrice pathway but still gave birth in the birth rooms.

ED AND MERRILY TIERNEY

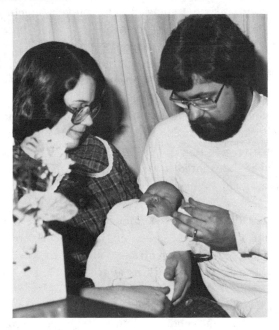

Ed: About a month and a half before Merrily was due with our first child, we began our Lamaze classes. We ended up taking one class, and then before we had any more Merrily ended up in the hospital and had the baby. We went in there with absolutely no experience whatsoever. The first class was nothing more than teaching us basic exercises.

Merrily: When we got to the hospital I was slightly hysterical because I thought something was wrong with the baby. At first I insisted that I had food poisoning and that I wasn't there to have the baby. The nurses were very helpful, and between contractions they taught me the breathing, for what that was worth. But it went fairly fast, and I had two paracervicals; the first one didn't take, and Dr. Sumner gave me another one.

Ed: The nurses were really very good. They were in every couple of minutes.

Merrily: That was 3 years ago when Kevin was born. With this pregnancy I had originally decided to take the private Lamaze classes and then I decided to just go to the hospital classes. I knew from the first time that the nurses would be helpful. (I can't say enough about the staff at Manchester.) So we took the two classes and had the tour of the hospital and, even though it was crowded, they worked individually with the couples. The first night was a double class and there were about 30 couples and three instructors. We learned breathing techniques and relaxation.

Ed: It's nice to go to the classes and learn all the breathing, but if you don't go home and practice, it's not going to help you very much. That was the key. I thought Merrily was a lot more controlled this time because of the breathing and knowing exactly what was going on.

Merrily: This time I actually waited at home a little bit. I was just sitting around, ready.

Ed: This time we were at the hospital for quite a while. Dr. Sumner came in about 4:30 when the nurse called him—it seemed like he got there awfully fast—and checked Merrily. She was dilated—9 centimeters, I think.

Merrily: I went from 6 to 9 very rapidly.

Ed: So he asked if she wanted to push, and they moved us down to the Gold Room at that point. We were there for quite a while, I guess about 45 minutes.

Merrily: I thought the pushing was a lot harder. I don't remember yelling for Ed to help me the first time, but this time I did. It was coming so rapidly and the pressure was so much stronger than with Kevin. It was a nice experience to have Brian stay with us afterward. He stayed with us about 45 minutes.

Ed: We were a lot less worried this time, too. With Kevin we didn't really get a chance to see him until about 12 hours after, whereas Brian stayed with us for quite a while, long enough for some pictures. He was nice and healthy . . . crying.

Although Ed and Merrily Tierney chose to attend the hospital prenatal classes and did not have a monitrice, their memories of their birth experience are warm and positive. To quote Merrily, "I can't say enough about the staff at Manchester." Staff attitudes are important to the birth experience; a warm environment alone will not make a humanistic birth.

JIM AND DIANE BEAULIEU

Diane and Jim are the parents of three boys. Their eldest son is 4 years old and was born at a hospital in a town close to Manchester. To prepare for this first birth, Diane and Jim had attended Lamaze classes. Unfortunately, their memories of this first birth are very unpleasant.

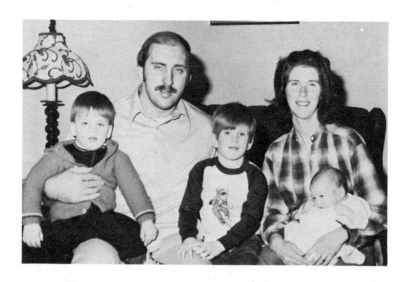

Diane: When we arrived at the hospital and the doors opened, all I heard was screaming women. There were two women in labor, and they were both screaming terribly. First they took me to this room I call the "torture chamber," and they sat me on this table; I don't think they even said hello to me. One nurse slapped a blood pressure cuff on my arm and took my blood pressure, which was 140/90. (I usually run a 100 to 110 blood pressure.) This elevated blood pressure upset them terribly. They didn't take into account that I was listening to screaming women, and was a little bit afraid too, since it was my first baby. Also, they had lost all of my records from the afternoon before, so when I got to the admitting room I had to sit there and be readmitted all over again. The first thing that they did was to draw up an injection of Vistaril, insisting that I had to have this Vistaril. Then they gave me a very large enema, something between 500 and 1000 cc's, and told me to sit on the toilet for 20 minutes. I was not to leave the toilet for anything! I think the hospital could have been burning down, and I would have had to sit there for 20 minutes. In the meantime, I don't even know where my husband was. He was not even allowed to come anywhere near me during this procedure. So next they prepped me and took me to the labor room, at which point I asked where my husband was. I told them that we had been to classes and were planning to be together. They said, "Where are your cards?" I said, "What cards?" They said that we should have been given cards. Well, I didn't have a card and I thought that for a minute they weren't going to let him stay.

In many hospitals in the United States, the prerequisite for admission to labor and delivery areas for fathers is proof of attendance at "acceptable" classes. There are not studies in the literature that substantiate the benefit of this practice. In fact, such requirements can serve to surround the entire birth experience with a sense of great mystery and impending peril. What is behind those hospital doors that is so special that a pass is needed to enter?

Luckily for Jim and Diane, the card requirement was waived after they convinced the staff that they had completed Lamaze classes. However, Jim never felt that he had a place in the experience.

Jim: I went through classes and all, granted, but I didn't have anything to do with this, especially from the father's point of view. "Step aside, stay out of our way. Go stand in the corner": that was their attitude.

This first labor progressed slowly with Diane feeling that everything which could have gone wrong did. She had an intravenous meperidine (Demerol), and hydroxyzine pamoate (Vistaril) injections, and "back labor."

Diane: I lost complete control. I had absolutely no control whatsoever. I was screaming. I was as bad as the women we heard when we first got off the elevator. Finally, about 7 A.M., they changed shifts and the day nurse came in. I was very discouraged at this point. The doctor did give me a paracervical, which gave me a break for an hour. I was able to doze off, and it was really very helpful. I don't think I could have made it if I hadn't had that paracervical. I was exhausted, drugged, and out of it. I had really had it. Then my water broke, and I went through the transition. When it was time to push, I was pushing well, and they moved me to the delivery room, and I got one more shot from the doctor into the IV. The whole delivery was kind of, well, I was awake, but it was sort of, well, I was really high. When David was born, he was very lethargic. It took a while for him to pink up. In fact, they gave him some oxygen. I'm sure it was from all that medication that I had.

The attitude and treatment of Jim as extraneous to the experience continued through labor and birth and into the postpartum period.

Diane: I lay in recovery—I was exhausted, I'll have to admit that. But I was in there with ladies who had cesareans. I felt very alone. I mean, you know, I had had the baby. Jim tried to come in and see me and they had an absolute coronary about it, literally, like he was going to infect the whole room. He was still in the clothes that he wore in the delivery room. I really don't know what the problem was. OK: that was David's birth, enough said about that experience. We didn't really know any better at that time. That was their idea in 1975 of Lamaze, or natural, or prepared birth, or whatever you want to call it.

Michael's birth was better. Three years had passed, and they were improving. We didn't go back for our review classes, but I very diligently read my book over again. This time they had my records. I still had to go to the "torture room," I still had the enema and the prep and the 20-minute wait and the IV, but luckily the IV went right in the first time around. I had said I would like to go into the Lamaze room, and they said that was fine but that it was being used. They told me to go into a regular labor room and that the woman was about ready to deliver and as soon as it was cleaned up they would transfer me. So I went in and lay down, and I was really feeling well. I was having contractions, but they weren't that bad. Everything was under control. The nurses wheeled over this machine and said, "We're going to hook you up to the fetal monitor." And I said, "Why?" "Well, because. . . it's our policy. We have them now, and we're going to use them." It's really silly because first they used the external. I'd look at the heartbeat and see "59," then "47." The nurse said, "Oh, that's not accurate." I said, "Well, what do you use it for if it's not accurate?" "Well, we can measure your contractions." I said, "Well, I can tell you that my contractions aren't doing that much." That was really silly. They were measuring something that was not accurate. What's the sense? Then the doctor came and broke my water and said, "Now we can hook you up to the internal monitor and that will be accurate." So they did their thing, and no sooner was I attached when they told me that the room was ready and I could walk down to it. We walked to the room. My contractions were not very strong, so the doctor said that since I was definitely in labor they would induce me. Instead of a 4- to 8-hour labor, I would have a 2- to 4-hour labor. They told me they were going to lunch and that they would start the induction when they came back. They went to lunch and Jim went to lunch, too. And I read my book. They started the induction at 1 o'clock.

Michael was delivered in the Lamaze room with anesthesia. He was a 9-pound baby, and after he was cleaned the nurses gave him to Diane to hold.

Jim: I wasn't able to hold him. They didn't let anybody hold him other than the mother. That was their policy. I was standing right there and didn't hold him. The option was never even offered to me.

For the birth of their third child, Jim and Diane chose Manchester Memorial Hospital.

Diane: This time around I decided I wanted to have the baby at Manchester, just because it was closer. I wanted to have my obstetrician in Manchester for the same reason.

Jim: We had just moved here when she was pregnant with Michael, so we remained with our original doctor for that birth. So being closer was really our reason for switching. After we went through it we realized that it was the best thing that we ever did. We weren't motivated to change because we were dissatisfied with our other experiences. We didn't know it would be any different anyplace else.

The Beaulieus are representative of many couples giving birth in the United States today. They were not aware of alternatives available to them for birth. Although they had prepared themselves for each birth by attending Lamaze classes and reading books, the environment in which their first experiences occurred was so controlled that they accepted it as the only reality.

John's birth was a marked contrast to the first two experiences.

Diane: When I got to the hospital my contractions were every 2 to 3 minutes. They were strong; I don't know if I was used to it or what, but it wasn't any big panic thing at all. We went in and were very pleasantly admitted. It was a very short thing. They asked me for a urine specimen. The admitting nurse told me that if I had a recent bowel movement, I wouldn't need an enema. I cracked up laughing. She must have thought I was insane. I said, "Yes, I did." So she said that it was only a Fleet enema anyway. I said, "You don't make me wait 20 minutes?" She said, "No." So I just got in bed and I was waiting for them to start attacking me, putting in needles or attaching things. Nothing happened. They got my husband a chair. They got me some ice. They told me they'd be in to check me every 10 to 15 minutes.

Jim: We couldn't believe it. We thought they must be slow and this must be one of these dead times. Surely, they don't do this to everybody. After awhile we started looking around, and it did seem to be the normal trend to be a little friendlier and let things go easier. No push and shove. . . definitely relaxed us.

Diane: There were two girls that had just delivered, so they were still being watched, and I was the only one in labor. All of a sudden I realized—you just know, especially when it's your third one—I just knew I was ready to deliver, so I asked Jim to go get the nurse quick. I said, "Just get the nurse. It's nothing you can do. Get the nurse in here. I have to be checked." She did find that I was fully dilated and ready to deliver. She asked me to give one push just to see and then said, "No more pushing, please," and everybody moved very rapidly, and they moved the stretcher in. There was really no problem. I was fully awake. Then they moved me down to the Lamaze room (the Gold Room) and called the doctor. He scrubbed up, and I gave a few pushes, and that was it. It was really very easy. They let me hold John right away, which was something that I had never done.

Jim: Since she had never done it, she was a little bit surprised. She said, "What is this?" He was all gray, and they put him right on her, and she goes, "Whooooooo."

Diane: Well, I did that because to me he didn't appear to be breathing. He was very dark, much darker than Michael, who was born screaming.

Jim: Because of all the fluid, and they hadn't cleaned him up yet.

Diane: I didn't realize that. There was a pocket of fluid when he was born and I had not seen that, and in those first seconds he did not appear to be breathing. He was very blue and I said, "Is he all right?" And Dr. Wheeler said, "Yes, he's fine." He suctioned him.

Jim: I got to hold the baby this time. It was quite a thrill. It was important and a lot different than before. It was more personal. Nothing really changes, but I had a real sense of satisfaction. It was nice to see that he was healthy and everything else. It was a moment that I'll remember for the rest of my life. I felt more a part of it. I wasn't just an observer.

Also, in the first few days after the birth, I spend a lot of time there. I got to hold him and watch him. The atmosphere was a lot easier. I didn't have to go looking for a gown in four closets and two hallways and everything else. The nurses show you what to do the first time, and after that you get your own gown and wash yourself. Also, our older ones came in to visit. They loved it. Michael wasn't too sure, but David, the 4-year-old, just loved it. Michael had been in the hospital with bronchitis a month before, and we think that had an adverse effect on him because he thought he was going to have to stay there again. He wasn't too sure. When he saw that I was going to take him back home again, then he wanted to see the baby. He knew he wasn't staying there. When we came back home, that's all they talked about for the rest of the day: "When's the baby coming home?" They were happy to see him. We were surprised, because for that age bracket we expected some jealousy. From the beginning they got the right idea and felt so good about it that half those feelings were wiped out before they got started. I'm no psychiatrist, but that's by opinion. Even today they don't have any animosity or hard feelings about the baby like I've seen in other homes. Other kids are completely turned-off, and it's not just because of the age group. David just loves to hold him, and Mike—as soon as he begins to cry—comes to get him. The whole thing seems to work out rather nice.

Diane and Jim's three birth experiences offer overwhelming evidence of the importance of staff attitudes to the quality of birth experiences. Their first birth was totally controlled and steeped in rigid policies and procedures. Although their second birth occurred in a birth room ("Lamaze room"), it was still a negative experience for them because of staff attitudes. Their third birth took place in a Manchester Memorial Hospital birth room without a monitrice in attendance. The difference in how they felt about that experience comes through in their interview loud and clear. Notice that they never even mention the room. It is the warm, accepting, supportive staff they remember.

BOB AND KATHLEEN BROWN

When their first child, Jayson, was 1 year old, Kathleen learned that she was $4^{1}/_{2}$ months pregnant. Although Kathleen and Bob had been planning on a home birth, complications required that Jayson be born in a hospital. Memories of that first birth were not pleasant, with Kathleen telling of feeling "cheated and robbed." Knowing that she was considered at risk and not a candidate for a home birth with this pregnancy, Kathleen talked of the birth center at Manchester Memorial Hospital as an "acceptable compromise."

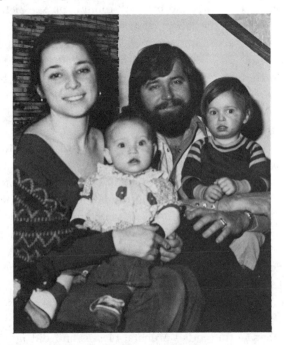

Kathleen: It was a blessing, an absolute blessing! To know that if you didn't have the option of a home birth, you could make it as comfortable as possible. I had a very good experience at Manchester. It as an excellent birth. I was fully prepared for it. In my own life I had become very strong, and I really wanted this child. I didn't know what the possibilities in the future would be for me to have any more children in our situation, and I really wanted her. The next thing I can relate is when labor began. It was a real nice day and we were getting along fine that day. I took a nap on the water bed we have and my son went down for a nap. I remember waking up and hearing a popping noise, and all of a sudden there was a flood on me. I thought the water bed had broken but found out my water had broken. The next thing I knew, I started the nice rhythm of labor and called to see what doctor was on call that night. I wanted to be attuned to whoever was on. I made some phone calls to someone to come to stay with Jayson. Bob had no phone where he was working so I had to find him, and we had to find a ride to the hospital. Things were moving very slowly. My labor progressed very nicely. My body cleansed itself, and I was able to control my breathing very well at home. It was very easy, and we got a friend to take me to the hospital.

People were very nice when we got into the admitting room. I thought I was going to go on into the birthing room. You see, I had no idea that I was going to stay in the labor room and transfer later on. A nurse came in the examined me and found out that I was 5 centimeters dilated and that's all I had to hear. The smile came on my face and I said, "I'm going to make it." My breathing was working really well and I didn't have anything for pain. The nurses were there and Bob finally got into the room, and we just sat around. Whenever I wanted to move or they wanted to examine me I was really in control of what I was doing. If I got too tense, I talked to someone to distract myself. Bob was really turned-on to me. Finally we started going down the hall, in fact, I got into a wheelchair, and went down the hall to the birthing room. We got there, and it was really very nice. I hadn't seen one before. I just got in there and felt very comfortable. Everyone was just hanging around in there watching me in labor. There was this beautiful big mirror so I wouldn't have to look in this tiny round one.

When Mandy was born, I was euphoric. She was fully aware. Her eyes were so bright, fully open. It was such a difference. We got to hold her and she looked right up at me. I tried nursing her, and I didn't even want to put her down. I just wanted to look at her. She was just bright-eyed and big-smiled.

Although they had not attended prenatal classes and did not have a monitrice in attendance, Kathleen and Bob found their birth experience in the Manchester birth room to be very satisfying.

Kathleen: I loved it there. I didn't want to go home. The food was so good at Manchester and the people were so nice. I wanted to get my nursing started and be comfortable before I did try to go home to two children relatively alone. When I was with Jayson after I had him, we didn't get along too well. It was very difficult to get adjusted to a brand new baby. Babies are difficult the first couple of months—not sleeping and so forth. When I had Mandy, it was a lot different, and I really feel that we made a really nice bond just by being together in the birthing room. I became a lot more tolerant of her because I was a lot closer to her than I was to Jayson. I'd do it again. I loved it! I don't think I'd have a birth at home. There's no reason not to go to the hospital. You won't have the rest afterwards if you have your baby at home, unless you have help. If there is a complication like I faced, there was no way I could have made it to the hospital in time. There would have been no way that I would be here, probably, to talk about it. I needed that rest after I had the baby. I needed someone to care for me. I think the idea of having a home birth will change as these places become more available.

A positive birth experience in a calm atmosphere became a reality for Kathleen and Bob in a hospital birth room. We will not know whether people now choosing home birth will accept hospital birth rooms as a compromise until such alternatives are available in every community. However, providing a hospital alternative to home birth is *not* the issue we are addressing. The issue is actually one of attitudinal change with the goal of providing a humanized hospital birth for *all families*.

REFERENCES

1. Adams, M., et al.: The confused patient: psychological responses in critical care units, Am. J. Nurs. 78:1504-1512, 1978.
2. Anderson, S. V.: Siblings at birth: a survey and study, Birth and Family J. 6(2):9,80-87, 1979.
3. Beck, N. C., and Hall, D. H.: Natural childbirth, a review and analysis, Am. J. Obstet. Gynecol. 52:371-379, 1978.
4. Brackbill, Y., Kane, T., Manniello, R. L., et al.: Obstetrical meperidine usage and assessment of neonatal status, Anesthesiology 40:116-120, Feb., 1974.
5. Brazelton, T. B.: Effect of prenatal drugs on the behavior of the neonate, Am. J. Psychiat. 126(9):95-100, 1970.
6. Brazelton, T. B.: Psychophysiologic relations in the neonate: effect of maternal medication, J. Pediatr. 58:513-518, 1961.
7. Caldeyro-Barcia, R.: The influence of the maternal position during the second stage of labor. In Simkin, P., and Reinke, C., editors: Kaleidoscope of childbearing preparation, birth and nurturing, Seattle, 1978, The Pennypress.
8. de Chateau, P.: The importance of the neonatal period for the development of synchrony in the mother-infant dyad, Birth and Family J. 4(1):10-22, 1977.
9. Flynn, A. M., Kelly, J., Hollins, G., and Lynch, P. F.: Ambulation in labour, Br. Med. J. 2:591, 1978.
10. Greenberg, M., and Morris, N.: Engrossment: the newborn's impact upon the father, Am. J. Orthopsychiatry 44:520-531, 1974.
11. Helsing, E.: Lactation education: the learning of the "obvious," Ciba Found. Symp. 45:215-230, 1976.
12. Highley, B. L., and Mercer, R. T.: Safeguarding the laboring woman's sense of control, Am. J. MCN 3(1):39-41, 1978.
13. Huttel, F. A., Mitchell, I., Fischer, W. M., and Meyer, A-E.: A quantitative evaluation of psychoprophylaxis in childbirth, J. Psychosom. Res. 16:81-92, 1972.
14. ICEA Conference, Washington, D.C., June, 1977.
15. Johnston, M.: Toward a culture of caring: children, their environment, and change, Am. J. MCN 4:210-214, 1979.
16. Klaus, M. H., and Kennell, J. H.: Maternal-infant bonding: the impact of early separation or loss on family development, St. Louis, 1976, The C. V. Mosby Co.
17. Klusman, L. E.: Reduction of pain in childbirth by the alleviation of anxiety during pregnancy, J. Consult. Clin. Psychol. 43(2):162-165, 1975.
18. Kron, R. E., and Goddard, K. E.: Newborn sucking behavior affected by obstetric sedation, Pediatrics 37:1012-1016, 1966.
19. Lederman, R., Lederman, E., Work, B., and McCann, D.: The relationship of maternal anxiety, plasma catecholamines, and plasma cortisol to progress in labor, Am. J. Obstet. Gynecol. 132:495-500, 1978.

20. McDonald, D. L.: Paternal behavior at first contact with the newborn in a birth environment without intrusions, Birth and Family J. 5(3):123-132, 1978.
21. Mendez-Bauer, C., et al.: Effects of standing position on spontaneous uterine contractility and other aspects of labor, J. Perinat. Med. 3:89-100, 1975.
22. Morris, N.: Human relations in obstetric practice, Lancet 1:913, 1960.
23. Norr, K. L., Block, C. R., Charles, A., et al.: Explaining pain and enjoyment in childbirth, J. Soc. Behav. 18(3):260-275, 1977.
24. Oster, C.: Sensory deprivation in geriatric patients, Am. Geriatr. Soc. 24(10):461-464, 1976.
25. Peterson, G. H., Mehl, L. E., and Leiderma, P. H.: The role of some birth-related variables in father attachment, Am. J. Orthopsychiatry 49(2):330-338, 1979.
26. Rubin, R.: Body image and self-esteem, Nurs. Outlook 16:20-23, June, 1968.
27. Scanlon, J. W., Brown, W. U., Weiss, J. B., et al.: Neurobehavioral responses of newborn infants after maternal epidural anesthesia, Anesthesiology 40(2):121-128, 1974.
28. Scott, J. R., and Rose, N. B.: Effect of psy-choprophylaxis (Lamaze preparation) on labor and delivery in primiparas, N. Engl. J. Med. 294(22):1205-1207, 1976.
29. Shelby, J. P.: Sensory deprivation, Image 10(2)49-55, 1978.
30. Skinner, B. F.: Beyond freedom and dignity, New York, 1971, Alfred A. Knopf.
31. Skinner, B. F.: The experimental analysis of behavior, Am. Sci. 45:347-371, 1957.
32. Skinner, B. F.: Science and human behavior, New York, 1953, Macmillan.
33. Standley, K., Soule, B., and Copans, S. A.: Dimensions of prenatal anxiety and their influence on pregnancy outcome, Am. J. Obstet. Gyneco. 135(22):22-26, 1979.
34. Tanzer, D. S.: The psychology of pregnancy and childbirth: an investigation of natural childbirth, unpublished Ph.D. dissertation, Brandeis University, Waltham, Mass., 1967.
35. Willmuth, L. R.: Prepared childbirth and the concept of control, JOGN Nurs. 4(5):38-41, 1975.
36. Wood, M.: Clinical sensory deprivation: a comparative study of patients in single care and two-bed rooms, J. Nurs. Adm. 7(10):28-32, 1977.

CHAPTER 4

Changing

The only stability possible is stability in motion.
John Gardner

FAMILY-CENTERED CARE

At the very heart of the Manchester experience and the other birth environments presented in this book is the concept of family-centered maternity/newborn care, which focuses on the physical, social, psychologic, and economic needs of the total family unit. The care given to this family includes them in decision making and planning, recognizing their individual needs, rights, and responsibilities. There is an emphasis on physical and emotional preparation for childbirth and parenthood, with a strong commitment to family values. To provide this care, a variety

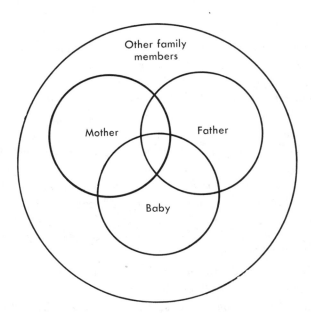

Fig. 4-1. The family.

of birth environments should be available, offering the family a choice while maintaining safety.

A joint position statement published by the Interprofessional Task Force on Health Care of Women and Children[8] endorsed the concept of family-centered care. For those hospitals choosing to offer family-centered maternity care, the task force recommended that:

1. Hospitals offer classes in preparation for birth for both mothers and fathers, including instruction on the role of men at birth
2. Ongoing education be made available to all hospital personnel involved in the family-centered program
3. Fathers remain with childbearing women as much as possible during the entire process
4. Parent-infant interaction immediately after birth be encouraged
5. Hospitals offer the option of using a homelike birthing room rather than a standard delivery room, which resembles a surgical facility
6. Provision be made for young children to visit their mothers and newborn siblings in the hospital
7. Hospitals develop programs for early discharge of mothers after birth, so the family can return to the more psychologically secure atmosphere of the home; this could include health professionals making home visits to families

The position statement emphasized, however, that the major change in maternity care needed to make family-centered care work is *attitudinal*. Providers of care for the childbearing family have a responsibility to ask themselves again and again, "Whose birth is this? To whom does the baby belong?"

STAFF

Changing staff attitudes may be the biggest challenge in converting hospitals from traditional maternity care to family-centered care. In many traditional settings the staff is in complete control, actively communicating to passive receivers of care. Orders are issued, and families are expected to follow submissively. Kalisch[9] terms this the active-passive continuum in which power is often invisible and most people are unaware of its existence. This can be a comfortable model for the health care provider, who is then the absolute authority and does not have to explain the "what" or "why" behind a policy. The statement, "You cannot visit your mother because that is hospital policy," is much easier for staff to say than explaining the scientific rationale for such policy.

Providing family-centered care means the staff has to assume a position of support vs. one of control. The childbearing family becomes a partner in decision making, with the staff offering expertise rather than authority. Interviews with professionals throughout the country who assumed this new role have disclosed their overwhelming satisfaction with it, although many of them will admit it was not a painless transition.

CONSUMERS

There is a great deal of consciousness-raising taking place among today's health care consumers. As part of this consumer movement, people are beginning to realize that they do not give up rights when they enter a hospital. In 1972 the American Hospital Association adopted "A Patient's Bill of Rights" as a national policy statement and distributed it to its member hospitals throughout the country.[10] Eight of the 12 rights relate to the patient's right to know or be informed. To be informed means to have the information necessary to given understanding consent to treatment. Informed consent implies participation in decisions. Also, the rights to know, to consent, to refuse consent, and to withdraw consent carry with them responsibilities that many of today's childbearing families are seeking.

More recently, a committee on patients' rights, headed by Doris and John Haire, published "The Pregnant Patient's Bill of Rights." "The Pregnant Patient's Responsibilities," was prepared by members of the International Childbirth Education Association. Both of these papers follow.

THE PREGNANT PATIENT'S BILL OF RIGHTS*

1. The Pregnant Patient has the right, prior to the administration of any drug or procedure, to be informed by the health professional caring for her of any potential direct or indirect effects, risks, or hazards to herself or her unborn or newborn infant which may result from the use of a drug or procedure prescribed for or administered to her during pregnancy, labor, birth, or lactation.
2. The Pregnant Patient has the right, prior to the proposed therapy, to be informed, not only of the benefits, risks, and hazards of the proposed therapy but also of known alternative therapy, such as available childbirth education classes, which could help to prepare the Pregnant Patient physically and mentally to cope with the discomfort or stress of pregnancy and the experience of childbirth, thereby reducing or eliminating her need for drugs and obstetric intervention. She should be offered such information early in her pregnancy in order that she may make a reasoned decision.
3. The Pregnant Patient has the right, prior to the administration of any drug, to be informed by the health professional who is prescribing or administering the drug to her that any drug which she receives during pregnancy, labor, and birth, no matter who or when the drug is taken or administered, may adversely affect her unborn baby, directly or indirectly, and that there is no drug or chemical which has been proven safe for the unborn child.

---

*Prepared by Doris Haire, Chairperson, Committee on Health Law and Regulation, International Childbirth Education Association, Inc.

4. The Pregnant Patient has the right, if Cesarean section is anticipated, to be informed prior to the administration of any drug, and preferably prior to her hospitalization, that minimizing her and, in turn, her baby's intake of nonessential preoperative medicine will benefit her baby.

5. The Pregnant Patient has the right, prior to the administration of a drug or procedure, to be informed if there is NO properly controlled follow-up research which has established the safety of the drug or procedure with regard to its direct and/or indirect effects on the physiological, mental, and neurological development of the child exposed, via the mother, to the drug or procedure during pregnancy, labor, birth, or lactation—(this would apply to virtually all drugs and the vast majority of obstetric procedures).

6. The Pregnant Patient has the right, prior to the administration of any drug, to be informed of the brand name and generic name of the drug in order that she may advise the health professional of any past adverse reaction to the drug.

7. The Pregnant Patient has the right to determine for herself, without pressure from her attendant, whether she will accept the risks inherent in the proposed therapy or refuse a drug or procedure.

8. The Pregnant Patient has the right to know the name and qualifications of the individual administering a medication or procedure to her during labor or birth.

9. The Pregnant Patient has the right to be informed, prior to the administration of any procedure, whether that procedure is being administered to her for her or her baby's benefit (medically indicated) or as an elective procedure (for convenience or teaching purposes).

10. The Pregnant Patient has the right to be accompanied during the stress of labor and birth by someone she cares for and to whom she looks for emotional comfort and encouragement.

11. The Pregnant Patient has the right after appropriate medical consultation to choose a position for labor and for birth which is least stressful to her baby and to herself.

12. The Obstetric Patient has the right to have her baby cared for at her bedside if her baby is normal and to feed her baby according to her baby's needs rather than according to the hospital regimen.

13. The Obstetric Patient has the right to be informed in writing of the name of the person who actually delivered her baby and the professional qualifications of that person. This information should also be on the birth certificate.

14. The Obstetric Patient has the right to be informed if there is any known or indicated aspect of her or her baby's care or condition which may cause her or her baby later difficulty or problems.

15. The Obstetric Patient has the right to have her and her baby's hospital medical records complete, accurate, and legible and to have their records, including Nurses' Notes, retained by the hospital until the child reaches at least the age of majority or, alternatively, to have the records offered to her before they are destroyed.

16. The Obstetric Patient, both during and after her hospital stay, has the right to have access to her complete hospital medical records, including Nurses' Notes, and to receive a copy upon payment of a reasonable fee and without incurring the expense of retaining an attorney.

   It is the obstetric patient and her baby, not the health professional, who must sustain any trauma or injury resulting from the use of a drug or obstetric procedure. The observation of the rights listed above will not only permit the obstetric patient to participate in the decisions involving her and her baby's health care, but will help to protect the health professional and the hospital against litigation arising from resentment or misunderstanding on the part of the mother.

THE PREGNANT PATIENT'S RESPONSIBILITIES*

In addition to understanding her rights the Pregnant Patient should also understand that she, too, has certain responsibilities. The Pregnant Patient's responsibilities include the following:

1. The Pregnant Patient is responsible for learning about the physical and psychological process of labor, birth, and postpartum recovery. The better informed expectant parents are the better they will be able to participate in decisions concerning the planning of their care.
2. The Pregnant Patient is responsible for learning what comprises good prenatal and intranatal care and for making an effort to obtain the best care possible.
3. Expectant parents are responsible for knowing about those hospital policies and regulations which will affect their birth and postpartum experience.
4. The Pregnant Patient is responsible for arranging for a companion or support person (husband, mother, sister, friend, etc.) who will share in her plans for birth and who will accompany her during her labor and birth experience.
5. The Pregnant Patient is responsible for making her preferences known clearly to the health professionals involved in her case in a courteous and cooperative manner and for making mutually agreed-upon arrangements regarding maternity care alternatives with her physician and hospital in advance of labor.
6. Expectant parents are responsible for listening to their chosen physician or midwife with an open mind, just as they expect him or her to listen openly to them.
7. Once they have agreed to a course of health care, expectant parents are responsible, to the best of their ability, for seeing that the program is carried out in consultation with others with whom they have made the agreement.
8. The Pregnant Patient is responsible for obtaining information in advance regarding the approximate cost of her obstetric and hospital care.
9. The Pregnant Patient who intends to change her physician or hospital is responsible for notifying all concerned, well in advance of the birth if possible, and for informing both of her reasons for changing.
10. In all their interactions with medical and nursing personnel, the expectant parents should behave toward those caring for them with the same respect and consideration they themselves would like.
11. During the mother's hospital stay, the mother is responsible for learning about her and her baby's continuing care after discharge from the hospital.
12. After birth, the parents should put into writing constructive comments and feelings of satisfaction and/or dissatisfaction with the care (nursing, medical, and personal) they received. Good service to families in the future will be facilitated by those parents who take the time and responsibility to write letters expressing their feelings about the maternity care they received.

*Prepared by members of the International Childbirth Education Association, Inc.

All the previous statements assume a normal birth and postpartum experience. Expectant parents should realize that, if complications develop in their cases, there will be an increased need to trust the expertise of the physician and hospital staff they have chosen. However, if problems occur, the childbearing woman still retains her responsibility for making informed decisions about her care or treatment and that of her baby. If she is incapable of assuming that responsibility because of her physical condition, her previously authorized companion or support person should assume responsibility for making informed decisions on her behalf.

Responsiveness to consumers' rights and responsibilities in the childbearing cycle requires dialogue. Open and honest communication between health care providers and childbearing families is vital. And since the capability of change is the basis for humanizing maternity care, an understanding of the change process is essential.

CHANGE

Frequently, when discussing concepts related to humanizing childbirth, hospital personnel will say, "We would like to promote family-centered care, but the other nurses (or our administrators or the physicians) are not interested." The reasons for resisting change are always numerous and very real, but for those who have recognized the need for change, there are ways of making things happen. In the following pages the change process is reviewed and strategies to promote change in maternity settings are presented.

Definitions

Change can be described as an alteration in the way an individual or group of individuals behave as a result of their redefining a situation.[21] In other words, change means creation of something different. Change can be neutral, can enrich and strengthen, or can destroy.[4] It can be planned or unplanned and either short or long term. However, planned change is more enduring. According to Bennis,[2] planned change is "a conscious, deliberate, and collaborative effort to improve the operation of a system, whether it be a self-system, social system, or cultural system, through the utilization of scientific knowledge." When change is too sudden or too drastic, individuals will often react with fear and psychologic or sometimes physical flight.[13]

Human behavior

Theories of social psychology and the behavioral sciences can be interwoven to explain human behavior in relation to change. For example, psychologists have found that, although it is an essential part of the process, insight itself does not produce change.[20] There are some theorists who envision behavior as a product of free will (internal control), whereas others see it as controlled by environment (external control). Still other theorists believe that individuals can be the product of conditioning and still be free to choose.[20]

Abraham Maslow[16] developed a motivation theory that is particularly useful when discussing change. According to Maslow, "all behavior is determined," and can be motivated in degrees from high to not at all. By conceptualizing the individual as an integrated whole, Maslow explained an individual's resistance to change as a by-product of a need for internal consistency. Basically, motivation theory structures human needs into a hierarchy, i.e., as one level is satisfied a higher level emerges, and so on. A brief summary of Maslow's hierarchy of human motivation follows.

5. Needs for self-actualization: what a person *can* be, he or she *must* be; desire for self-fulfillment, to become everything that one is capable of becoming
4. Esteem needs
   a. Desire for strength, achievement, adequacy, mastery, and competence; for confidence, independence and freedom
   b. Desire for reputation and prestige (respect or esteem from others), status, dominance, recognition, importance, or appreciation
3. Belongingness and love needs: involve both giving and receiving love
2. Safety needs: preference for familiar rather than unfamiliar, known rather than unknown; emphasize job protection
1. Basic physiologic needs: food, water, elimination, and rest

Since attitudes and behavior are related in complex ways, for change to be meaningful, attitudes, values, or beliefs must be changed. According to Rokeach,[18] "An attitude is a relatively enduring organization of beliefs around an object or situation predisposing one to respond in some preferential manner."

Although attitudes are learned rather than innate, not all attitudes are based on rational beliefs. Beliefs are cognitive perceptual responses that can describe, evaluate, and advocate action with respect to an object or situation. Beliefs can be conscious or unconscious and can be inferred from what a person says or does. Verbal statements of belief are preceded by the phrase, "I believe that . . . ."[18]

Some factors that contribute to beliefs include (1) cultural background, (2) observations, (3) feedback from others, (4) socialization, (5) education, and, of course, (6) the media.[22]

Values are enduring beliefs that certain ways of behaving or life-styles are preferable to alternative modes.[18] An individual's value system is a learned organization of rules that enable the person to make choices which result in overt actions or behavior.

In summary, attitudes have affective, learned, and behavioral components and are susceptible to change.

Theories of attitudinal and behavioral change. Zimbardo and colleagues[22] have identified five major theories of attitudinal and behavioral change. Very briefly, these include the following approaches*:

1. Yale attitude change approach basically indicates that attitudes are changed by changing beliefs. Those responsible for initiating this change must be credible, have expertise, and be trustworthy.
2. Group dynamics approach, developed by Kurt Lewin at the University of Michigan, indicates that the group norm can influence behavior. Attitudes people feel are their own often come from the groups to which they belong.
3. Cognitive dissonance theory, from the work of Leon Festinger in 1957, proposes that individuals cannot tolerate discrepancies in their cognitive systems. For example, when a person smokes cigarettes although he knows such action can cause lung cancer and heart disease, that person's behavior is inconsistent, or dissonant, with the knowledge held. It will be necessary for the individual to reduce the dissonance by changing behavior (stopping smoking), changing internal environment (adopting attitudes such as "only other people die"), or altering the external environment (e.g., removing warnings on cigarette packs).
4. Attribution theory explains actions by oversimplifying the real causes for behavior, as when someone says, "I cheated because I'm no good."
5. Social learning theory proposes that behavioral change is learned and that the environment can control how individuals behave. If behavior produces positive consequences, that behavior will recur. However, if behavior results in negative consequences, the same behavior is unlikely to recur.

Change agent

In the early literature[14] on change, a "change agent" referred to an outside skilled helper who would effect change in an organization. Today the change agent role has been broadened to include any individual or group, inside or outside the organization, who attempts to effect change.[2]

Communities

Since organizations function within communities, a look at the construct of communities is necessary before examining organizations. Iannaccone and Lutz[7] describe communities in terms of a sacred-secular continuum construct.

Sacred community	as opposed to	Secular community
Static		Lacks stability—in constant flux
Will accept some changes		Expert's testimonial = leverage for innovation
Introduce as slight modifications of accepted techniques instead of a new way		Written word = basis for innovation
Experience is best teacher—one's intimate must report successful experience with the innovation		The use of an innovation by competitors increases its chance of adoption

*From Zimbardo, P. G., Ebbesen, E., and Maslach, C.: Influencing attitudes and changing behavior, ed. 2, © 1979, Addison-Wesley Publishing Co., Inc., Paraphrase of pp. 56-84. Reprinted with permission.

Table 5. Characteristics of static vs. future-oriented organizations*

Dimensions	Characteristics	
	Static organizations	Future-oriented organizations
Structure	Rigid: permanent committees, reverence for constitution and bylaws, tradition Hierarchical: chain of command Role definitions narrow Property bound and restricted	Flexible: temporary task force, readiness to change constitution and bylaws, depart from tradition Linking: functional collaboration Role definitions broad Property mobile and regional
Atmosphere	Internally competitive Task centered, reserved Cold, formal, aloof	Goal oriented People oriented, caring Warm, informal, intimate

Management and philosophy	Controlling: coercive power
	Cautious, low risk
	Errors: to be prevented
	Emphasis on personnel selection
	Self-sufficient: closed system concerning resources
	  Emphasis on conserving resources
	Low tolerance for ambiguity
		Releasing: supportive power
		Experimental, high risk
		Errors: to be learned from
		Emphasis on personnel development
		Interdependent: open system concerning resources
		  Emphasis on developing and using resources
		High tolerance for ambiguity

Decision making and policy making	High participation at top, low at bottom Clear distinction between policy making and execution Decision making by legal mechanisms Decisions treated as final	Relevant participation by all those affected Collaborative policy making and execution Decision making by problem solving Decisions treated as hypotheses to be tested
Communication	Restricted flow, constipated One way—downward Feelings repressed or hidden	Open flow: easy access Two way—upward and downward Feelings expressed

*Reproduced with permission from Lippitt, G. L.: Hosp. Prog. **54:**55–64, June, 1973. Copyright 1973 by The Catholic Health Association. Chart developed by Malcolm Knowles.

The sacredness or secularity of a community affects the methods by which change can take place. For planning change, Iannaccone and Lutz[7] recommend first using techniques known to work in sacred communities. Techniques for implementing change in secular communities can be used as a last resort.

Organizations

Since an institution is originally established to preserve a change, it resists further change by its very nature. Unfortunately, the longer such an institution survives, the more obsolete what it is preserving becomes. John Gardner[4] emphasized the need for renewal in both individuals and institutions when he observed:

> When organizations and societies are young, they are flexible, fluid, and not yet paralyzed by rigid specialization and willing to try anything once. As the organization or society ages, vitality diminishes, flexibility gives way to rigidity, creativity fades, and there is a loss of capacity to meet challenges from unexpected directions. . . . In the ever-renewing society (or organization), what matures is a system or framework within which continuous innovation, renewal, and rebirth can occur.

Aging organizations, in their development of defenses against new ideas, often exhibit a preoccupation with methods, policies, procedures, and techniques. Within such organizations, the most powerful forces producing rigidity are often those with vested interests in maintaining the status quo.[4]

Most hospitals are bureaucratic organizations in which physicians exert a great deal of influence. Bureaucracies are characterized by a well-defined chain of command, with communication tending to flow from the top downward. Also, in such organizations there is a controlling system of rules and procedures to deal with work activities. Labor is divided according to specialization, and the reward structure is based on technical competence. The leadership style, being autocratic, tends to foster impersonality in human relations.[1,19] In Gordon Lippitt's[15] model for describing and dissecting an organization the characteristics of static organizations are descriptive of many hospitals (Table 5).

RESISTANCE TO CHANGE

Resistance to change can be caused by threats to the traditional values of the group and by change occurring too quickly.[11] Professional and quasi-professional groups bind people together and may resist change in the organization at large if it is seen as a threat to the group.[5]

The characteristics of people who do well within bureaucracies include loyalty to the system and acceptance of the legitimacy of rules and of external control and supervision. Often these people seek promotion based on allegiance to organizational policies and requirements. Historically, nursing and medical training indoctrinated students into the bureaucratic structure.[1] Consequently many of the personnel in positions of authority in hospitals have primary allegiance to the organization and resist change in its structure, no matter what the reason.

Strategies

There are many models of the change process, but perhaps the most succinct is the work of Ronald Havelock.[6] According to his model, it is essential in the beginning to build a good, trusting *relationship* between the change agent and the people involved in the change. Human needs of those involved must be taken into account, since change is more acceptable when it is understood and does not threaten. Also, change is more successful when those affected have helped to create it. In building this relationship, the problems to solve must be identified.

In the *diagnosis* of the problem, *acquisition* of relevant resources can be accomplished by interviewing individuals and groups. There are usually problem vocalizers and key informants. Also, observation as a participant or an observer and data collecting from print resources and files are important. Collection of these data from relevant resources will ultimately lead to well-defined change goals and problems. (It is important to distinguish problems from symptoms.)

Choosing the situation to begin the change process then follows from (1) deriving implications from the research, (2) generating a range of solution ideas, (3) feasibility testing, and (4) adoption.

Gaining *acceptance* is complex and involves people seeing for themselves some benefits in the change. As acceptance is gained, the change is stabilized. For a change to be long term, it must generate *self-renewal*, with provisions made for periodic review and revision. Continuing reward and satisfaction are very important. An overemphasis can be placed on changing individuals without considering the larger system (community and organization).

An excellent illustration of a plan using Havelock's strategies can be found in a description[3] of a major change in the maternity program at the Toledo Hospital in northwest Ohio, developed over a 5-year period. Principal change agent was a nursing staff member serving as Perinatal Supervisor at the time. Implicit in the experience was a trusting *relationship* between the change agent and administration and medical staff. This relationship was maintained by preparing and presenting to administration and medical staff written proposals as each phase of the program was ready for implementation.

In *diagnosing* the problem, *acquisition* of relevant resources included evaluation of the existing program, which involved listening to consumer requests for services not provided by the hospital maternity program. Many consumers wanted prenatal education and a more homelike delivery atmosphere and were threatening to patronize other hospitals for childbirth services. Since most American hospitals are big business, threats to remove sources of revenue often serve as catalysts for change.

The next step was to share an assessment summary with both hospital and nursing administration, as well as medical staff. Need for change was clearly identified by the assessment summary.

In *choosing* the situation in which to begin the change process, the agent initiated simple changes first. Gradual introduction to the new philosophy was accomplished by hospital in-service programs, conferences, and workshops. An instructor was hired to teach hospital-based prenatal classes, with physicians and nurses on staff made aware of class content. As each change was made, all staff members were included, recognizing that attitudinal change had to parallel changes in policy.

It was a slow process, but it worked. *Acceptance* happened as staff members experienced intangible rewards in the form of patient satisfaction. *Self-renewal* was obvious in plans for expansion of the program. Almost 5 years after the change process began, family-centered care was offered to all families, and the goal was a reality.

Paukert's[17] description of the process of implementing family-centered maternity care at Chicago Lying-In Hospital is another helpful illustration of the change process. Since the nursing department was fairly autonomous, the nursing administrators were able to change policies necessary to implement family-centered care without obtaining approval from external sources. However, it appears that a trusting *relationship* existed between nursing, medical staff, and hospital administration, because a collaborative approach was established. Nursing kept these other areas informed, consulted with them, and implemented their feedback whenever possible.

The change agent was a clinical specialist who assumed primary responsibility for this major change. To avoid staff resentment, this person was given line authority for the postpartum and normal nursery areas, where implementation of family-centered maternity care was a priority in the beginning.

Diagnosing the need for change came through *acquisition* of relevant factors, which included statistical data. It was noted that the perinatal mortality in the area served by the Chicago Lying-In Hospital was higher than the national average (CLI = 38/1000 births, national average = 20/1000 births). There was also a high incidence of failure-to-thrive infants being admitted to the University of Chicago Children's Hospital. With this information, nursing administrators decided that family-centered maternity care could improve these poor statistics by improving the mother's caretaking behavior.

Careful preliminary planning was done, and after some initial problems with staff resistance were solved a reasonable timetable for implementation was established. In *choosing* where to begin the implementation of change, the clinical specialist divided her overall goals into four steps.

Strategies for overcoming staff resistance included group process, in-service workshops, option to transfer out of the unit, and open communication. Since implementation occurred in stages, *acceptance* came as it was gradually demonstrated to the staff that family-centered maternity care worked.

That *self-renewal* was occurring is seen in the results of a questionnaire given to 32 staff members on both day and night shifts. In 27 questionnaires completed, 63% of the staff said that they did not want to return to traditional care and 11% had no preference. That's not 100%, but it is well on the way.

In these illustrations, the people involved recognized a need to change, and Havelock's model was effective. When people are not committed to change or change must be immediate, other strategies are necessary.

Zaltman and Duncan[21] place strategies for change into five groupings:

A. Reeducative strategies are feasible, other things being equal, when change does not have to be immediate.
   1. First establish awareness of need.
   2. If change requires high degree of commitment, reeducative strategies alone will not work.
   3. Are essential when change involves radical departure from past practice.
B. Persuasive strategies exert greater pressure toward a particular attitudinal and/or behavioral change than educative strategies and less than power strategies.
   1. Use when people not committed to change.
   2. Use when problem not recognized or considered important.
   3. Are especially effective in combating resistance to change.
C. Power strategies
   1. Are unlikely to increase commitment.
   2. Are desirable if decision-making process slow and change must be immediate.
   3. Can work before resistance can be mobilized; involve coercion to obtain compliance.
D. Facilitative strategies
   1. People recognize problem—willing to be involved in self-help.
   2. Create awareness of availability of assistance.
E. Multiple strategies are a combination of two or more.

Regardless of the strategy used, it is essential to include all those involved when planning change. As Irene Lee[12] said, "Nobody drills a hole in the boat if he's in it."

REFERENCES

1. Ashley, J.: Hospitals, paternalism, and the role of the nurse, New York, 1977, Teachers College Press.
2. Bennis, W. Q., Benne, K. D., and Chin, R., editors: The planning of change: readings in the applied behavioral sciences, New York, 1961, Holt, Rinehart, & Winston.
3. Candy, M.: Birth of a comprehensive family-centered maternity program, JOGN Nurs. 8(2):80-84, 1979.
4. Gardner, J.: Self-renewal: the individual and the innovative society, New York, 1963, Harper & Row Publishing Co.
5. Grossman, L.: The change agent, New York, 1974, Amacom.

6. Havelock, R. G.: The change agent's guide to innovation in education, Englewood Cliffs, N.J., 1973, Educational Technology Publications.
7. Iannaccone, L., and Lutz, F. W.: Politics, power and policy: the governing of local school districts, Columbus, Ohio, 1970, Charles E. Merrill Publishing Co.
8. Interprofessional Task Force on Health Care of Women and Children: Joint position statement on the development of family-centered maternity/newborn care in hospitals, Chicago, June, 1978.
9. Kalisch, B. J.: Of half gods and mortals; Aesculapian authority, Nurs. Outlook 23(1):22-28, 1975.
10. Kelly, L. Y.: The patient's right to know, Nurs. Outlook 24(1):26-32, 1976.
11. Knezevich, S. T.: Administration of public education, ed. 3, New York, 1975, Harper & Row Publishing Co.
12. Lee, I. M.: Cope with resistance to change, Nurs. '73 3(3):7, 1973.
13. Likert, R.: New patterns of management, New York, 1961, McGraw-Hill Book Co.
14. Lippett, R.: The dynamics of planned change, New York, 1958, Harcourt-Brace.
15. Lippitt, G. L.: Hospital organization in the post-industrial society, Hosp. Prog. 54:55-64, June, 1973.
16. Maslow, A. H.: Motivation and personality, New York, 1954, Harper & Row Publishing Co.
17. Paukert, S. E.: One hospital's experience with implementing family-centered maternity care, JOGN Nurs. 8(6):351-358, 1979.
18. Rokeach, M.: Beliefs, attitudes and values, a theory of organization and change, San Francisco, 1970, Tossey-Bass, Inc.
19. Sasmor, J.: Childbirth education: a nursing perspective, New York, 1979, John Wiley & Sons.
20. Wheelis, A.: How people change, New York, 1973, Harper & Row Publishing Co.
21. Zaltman, G., and Duncan, R.: Strategies for planned change, New York, 1977, John Wiley & Sons.
22. Zimbardo, P. G., Ebbesen, E., and Maslach, C.: Influencing attitudes and changing behavior, ed. 2, Reading, Mass., 1979, Addison-Wesley Publishing Co.

SUGGESTED READING

Kimbrough, R. B.: Political power and educational decision-making, Chicago, 1964, Rand McNally & Co.

CHAPTER 5

Nursing

FRAGMENTATION OF CARE

Hospital organization, we know, makes constant attendance upon all women in labor extremely difficult, but within the last 5 years some few understanding professors have instituted labor sisters who never leave the patients alone. We sympathize with all who work in hospitals where such service is hampered by inadequate provision of staff and space for individual attention during all phases of labor, but in private practice it is one of the main sources from which troubles in labor arise. Therefore, I repeat, take personal interest in your patient and remember that no woman should ever suffer the mental (and therefore physical) agony of loneliness whilst she is in labor.[14]

Dr. Grantly Dick-Read[14] wrote this in 1944 when he described how "frightful loneliness can be" in his book *Childbirth Without Fear*. In the more than 3 decades since Dr. Read wrote so poignantly on the "crime of enforced loneliness" in labor, research has given evidence that he was right.[6,8,13]

And yet, when visiting labor and delivery areas of hospitals today, one can still find many women laboring alone, frightened and lonely. From time to time a nurse may check on their progress, offer support, and then go on to another woman or other responsibilities. There is often the problem of too much to do with too few nurses to do it. But closer observation of these situations may find staff practicing avoidance behavior, such as refilling supply cupboards, sorting chart forms, and making gauze sponges. Even closer observation may find staff simply avoiding the laboring women except for routine assessments. Supporting women and their families in labor day after day is exhausting and depleting work. In the traditional routinized and compartmentalized maternity system, there are few rewards for nurses. Nurses who interact with women only for labor and birth, the postpartum period, or nursery care are working with just one piece of the birth experience. Such fragmentation of care does not permit the nurse to see the experience as a whole or the results of the work of all involved. In other words, for nurses functioning in compartments, there is no final closure or resolution of these pieces of the birth experience. Is it any wonder that nurses who function only in labor and delivery sometimes equate themselves with surgical nurses, that nurses who function only in newborn nurseries often speak of the babies as their own, or that nurses who provide care only on postpartum units are often hesitant to rotate to labor and delivery because of their lack of understanding of what happens there? As long as nurses continue to offer their skilled professional care in fragments, family-centered care will be only a dream.

In family-centered maternity care, ideally, mothers and babies should have the option of being together in the same room post partum. Babies may be returned to a central nursery whenever the family or staff deem this necessary. Fathers are not considered visitors and may come and go as is convenient for the family. Visitors may be restricted in both number and time or excluded completely. Sibling visiting is possible either in the mother's room or in a special sibling visiting room. Nursing staff members are assigned to care for mother/baby units, and a thorough program of teaching to facilitate infant-care skills and parenting is emphasized.

REDEFINITION OF NURSING ROLES

How can nursing be used to reduce the fragmentation of maternity care? The range of possibilities is limited only by one's imagination.

Monitrice

The monitrice concept, as implemented at Manchester Memorial Hospital, is an ideal solution to staffing hospital maternity units. It uses an experienced maternity nurse trained in the psychoprophylactic method (monitrice) to support the woman and her family on a one-to-one basis through labor and delivery (Fig. 5-1). Because the monitrice may also teach Lamaze classes in preparation for birth, there is continuity between antepartal and intrapartal nursing. With a group of monitrices available, a hospital literally has an on-call staff of private duty nurses for labor and delivery. The monitrice is part of a team made up of regular nursing and medical staff. Nursing staff may assume responsibility for admission and support until the monitrice arrives, and then resume responsibility for newborn and postpartum care. Of course, monitrice and staff work together as a team in case of complications or situations requiring surgical intervention. Maternity nurses who choose to work only a few days a week or full time can find the role of monitrice very rewarding. Nurses who organize a private monitrice program are in private practice, receiving a fee for services from the families served.[9] Each monitrice may have her own professional insurance, or the group may purchase insurance coverage.

Some institutions may find it easier to subdivide the role of the monitrice into two separate functions: (1) a labor attendant who is not an RN but is knowledgeable and experienced in prepared childbirth and is highly motivated to provide contin-

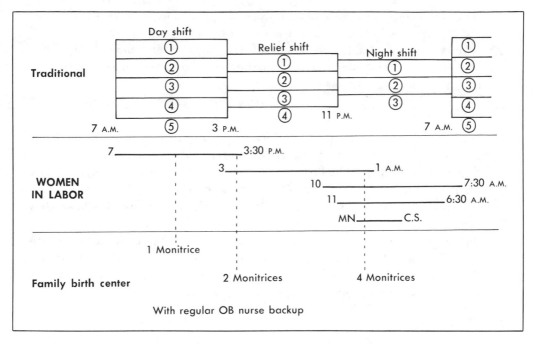

Fig. 5-1. Maternity nursing services, traditional vs. family birth center.

uous one-to-one emotional support; and (2) the obstetric nurse who monitors the mother's and the fetus' vital signs but is otherwise free to leave the room to perform other duties. Thus childbirth educators who are not nurses are not denied the opportunity to share in the drama of birth.

On-call staffing

A similar solution to the unpredictable availability of hospital maternity services is on-call staffing. Kowalski[10] described the use of two-nurse teams to carry a case load of patients through prenatal clinic, intrapartum, and postpartum periods. Upon admission of a patient in labor, the nurse on call goes to the hospital to provide care throughout labor and delivery. According to Kowalski, "Each nurse is scheduled to be in the obstetric clinic 16 hours per week and on call for labors every other 24 hours and every other weekend." To ensure continuity of care, each team nurse tries to see every patient at least twice for antepartum care. Scheduling is such that each team nurse works an average of 40 hours per week. Regular staffing is modified, but the need to care for six or more women in labor is less frequent than before on-call staffing. Both patients and nurses report satisfaction with the on-call system.[10] In a service such as this, the nurse is employed by the fee-for-service clinic that provides the maternity care.

Many hospitals with birth rooms also use on-call staffing, developing a call list from staff nurses who volunteer or from nurses who wish to work only on call. These nurses provide one-to-one nursing care throughout labor and delivery. They are considered hospital employees, are paid by the hospital, and are covered by the hospital's professional practice insurance.

Shared Beginnings

In the San Francisco Bay area, the *Shared Beginnings* nursing care program is a variation of on-call staffing.[7] It involves a group of nurses who are on call for the birth experience itself and the first 4 to 6 hours after birth to provide nursing care and facilitate parent-infant bonding. They also make follow-up telephone calls after hospital discharge and follow-up home visits to the family, if requested. Since they are essentially private duty nurses, families pay them directly.

On-call programs offer personalized care and take the burden of heavy census periods off regular staff. However, if the on-call nurses are seen as outsiders, they could represent a threat to regular staff. Group meetings attended by both staff and on-call nurses are essential to keep communication open.

Flexible staffing

Rotation of nursing staff through all areas of maternity care systems provides flexibility in staffing and certainly more relevant care. It means involvement in the maternity cycle instead of in segments of it, i.e., family-centered care. Such rotation may begin with nursing staff teaching prenatal classes and ends with the same staff making postpartum home visits.

Primary nursing is designed to replace team or functional nursing by assigning accountability for 24-hour care to one RN for specific patients throughout their hospital stay. This concept of nursing care involves patients and their families in their own care and places the nurses in the role of patient advocate.[4] Primary nursing offers individualized continuity of care in which technicians and trained paraprofessionals take over nonnursing duties.[1] It has been shown to be cost efficient and rewarding for staff, as well as patients.[2,5]

Family-centered maternity nursing is modified primary nursing. It involves as many staff nurses as possible teaching prenatal classes in the home or hospital. In this way, families meet interact, and establish rapport with their nurses before delivery day.

The staff consists of nurses and paraprofessionals who rotate through all areas of the maternity unit. Thus a nurse may be on duty in the labor area (birth room or traditional delivery room) on Monday and in the postpartum area on Tuesday. Ideally, rotation patterns would be circular, changing daily, so that there would be a high probability of one nurse following a family throughout their hospital stay.

However, if the facility and staff are very large, rotation may have to be on a weekly basis.

This flexible staffing plan provides the same continuity of care that is stressed in primary nursing. With the same nurses interacting with families beginning with prenatal education through birth and postpartum, optimal benefits can be gained.[2]

Home visits

The first 2 weeks after birth have been identified as a major period of crisis for family adjustment.[3] This is an ideal time for nurses to offer the family support and education. Provision for hospital staff nurses to make home visits is an extension of family-centered nursing care; it is nursing care come full circle. Although postpartum home visits are a part of alternative birth center programs in many hospitals, in others they are a part of family-centered care. Nursing staff are usually paid on a fee-for-visit basis by the employing hospital.

Other provisions for follow-up care include home visits by visiting nurses in the community, follow-up telephone calls, and community support groups.

Paraprofessionals

Imaginative and innovative research is needed to create educational programs for health paraprofessionals who can work with nurses. Such paraprofessionals could teach prepared childbirth classes, provide prenatal counseling, offer support during labor, and work in the home during the postpartum period providing necessary physical and emotional support to the family. They could be valuable liaisons with health professionals, closing the gap where professional staff shortages exist.

Special nursing roles

Certified nurse-midwives, nurse practitioners, and clinical specialists have important roles in the maternity team. However, a discussion of these roles is beyond the scope of this book. For those interested in the concept of the health care team, see "Joint Statement on Maternity Care" (1971) and "Supplementary Statement" (1975) in Appendix A.

OUTLINE FOR IN-SERVICE EDUCATION PROGRAM

For nurses to function in family-centered maternity care, they need skills in each of those areas which have traditionally been compartmentalized: antepartum, intrapartum, and postpartum periods, and newborn nursery. Separate classes offered in each sphere of experience allow staff to select those where they are weakest.

If nurses are to be involved with families choosing prepared childbirth methods, it is essential that they understand the methods used in their community. Dr.

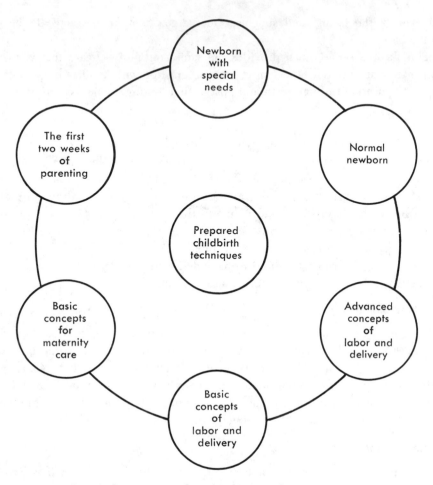

Fig. 5-2. Content areas for an in-service education program.

Lamaze,[11] in describing the necessary conditions for painless childbirth, clearly identified staff requirements as follows:

This is the essential pillar on which the success of childbirth without pain rests.

It is imperative to have an educated staff, whatever its status.

Any person intimately or remotely concerned with the unit working towards painless childbirth must be educated, as this person will affect the parturients. Each person plays a part in creating the atmosphere, the tone that must prevail in the Maternity Unit. The four essential qualities are:

1. Gentle behavior and voice
2. Kindness of action
3. Understanding, which always brings one nearer the woman
4. Calmness, which does away with impatience

An in-service program might include content areas as diagramed in Fig. 5-2, and is outlined below. Because of regional variations in standards of nursing care, only very broad and simple outlines are suggested here. These are simply a skeleton on which more comprehensive outlines can be built to meet individual nursing needs. Each major content area is divided into four separate learning sessions.

A. Basic concepts for maternity care
  1. Anatomy and physiology of pregnancy
    a. Female reproductive system
    b. Female pelvis
    c. Conception
    d. Physiologic adaptations to pregnancy
  2. Fetal development
    a. Implantation
    b. Embryonic period
    c. Fetal period
    d. Placenta
    e. Teratogens
  3. Paternal and maternal needs in pregnancy
    a. Nutritional
    b. Emotional
    c. Sexual
    d. Physical
    e. Educational
      (1) Prenatal education
      (2) Genetic counseling
  4. Nursing care in pregnancy
    a. Assessments
    b. Interventions
    c. Evaluation
B. Basic concepts of labor and delivery
  1. Anatomy and physiology of labor
    a. Hormone levels
    b. Uterine muscle
    c. Mechanism of labor and delivery
      (1) Passenger
      (2) Passageway
      (3) Powers
      (4) Psyche
  2. Paternal and maternal needs in labor and delivery
    a. Normal labor patterns
    b. Physical needs
    c. Emotional needs
    d. Roles
  3. Nursing care in labor and delivery
    a. Assessments
    b. Interventions
    c. Evaluation
  4. Introduction to risk screening
    a. Classification
    b. Screening tools
    c. Premature labor
      (1) Etiology
      (2) Management
      (3) Anticipatory nursing for mother, father, and baby
C. Advanced concepts of labor and delivery
  1. Abnormal labor
    a. Patterns
    b. Induction and augmentation
    c. Monitoring
    d. Cesarean births
    e. Nursing assessments and interventions
  2. Hypertensive states of pregnancy
    a. Toxemias
    b. Chronic hypertensive states
    c. Nursing assessments and interventions for toxemia and hypertensive women in pregnancy, labor, and delivery
    d. Anticipatory nursing measures for newborn of hypertensive mothers
  3. The pregnant diabetic
    a. Classifications
    b. Medical management
    c. Fetal implications
    d. Nursing assessments and interventions with pregnant diabetic, fetus, and newborn
  4. Bleeding in pregnancy and labor
    a. Early bleeding problems
    b. Placenta previa
    c. Abruptions
    d. Nursing assessments and interventions in bleeding problems during pregnancy, labor, and birth

D. Normal newborn
  1. The newborn baby
    a. Initiation of respiration
    b. Temperature regulation
    c. Nutritional needs
    d. Physical needs
    e. Daily observation and nursing care
  2. Perinatal assessment of maturation
    a. Average for gestational age
      (1) Identification
      (2) Statistics
      (3) Nursing management
    b. Small for gestational age
      (1) Identification
      (2) Statistics
      (3) Nursing management
    c. Large for gestational age
      (1) Identification
      (2) Statistics
      (3) Nursing management
  3. Bonding
    a. Theory
    b. Implications
    c. Nursing interventions
  4. Minor disorders of the newborn
    a. Physiologic jaundice
    b. Skin rashes
    c. Common variations from normal
    d. Nursing intervention
E. Newborn with special needs
  1. Identificaton of infant at risk
    a. Classifications
      (1) Statistics
      (2) Case finding
    b. Interventions
    c. Nursing care
  2. Respiratory problems
    a. Asphyxia neonatorum
      (1) Mild asphyxia
        (a) Cause
        (b) Signs
        (c) Treatment
        (d) Nursing interventions
      (2) Severe asphyxia
        (a) Cause
        (b) Signs

        (c) Treatment
        (d) Nursing care
    b. Respiratory distress syndrome
      (1) Etiology
      (2) Management
      (3) Nursing care
  3. Infections
    a. Types
      (1) Umbilical infections
        (a) Cause
        (b) Signs
        (c) Management
      (2) Urinary tract infection
        (a) Cause
        (b) Signs
        (c) Management
      (3) Generalized sepsis in the newborn; nursing interventions
      (4) Gastroenteritis
      (5) Respiratory tract infections
    b. Prevention and control
  4. Disorders
    a. Metabolic
    b. Neurologic
F. The first 2 weeks of parenting
  1. Physiology of the postpartum period
    a. Involution
    b. Physiologic changes in body systems
    c. Lactation
    d. Complications
      (1) Hemorrhage
      (2) Infections
      (3) Thromboemboli
  2. Paternal and maternal needs
    a. Taking-in
    b. Taking hold
    c. Letting go
    d. Breast or bottle feeding
    e. Emotional support
  3. Nursing care
    a. Assessments
    b. Interventions
    c. Evaluation
  4. Parenting
    a. Roles
    b. Responsibilities
    c. Sexuality

G. Prepared childbirth techniques
  1. Theories of childbirth education
    a. Historical background
    b. Description of methods currently used
      (1) Lamaze
      (2) Bradley
      (3) Read
      (4) Others
    c. Principles and objectives of childbirth education in general
    d. The participants in prepared childbirth
      (1) Woman in labor
      (2) Father or other support person
      (3) Medical team
    e. The basic prepared childbirth course
  2. Support of the couple in early labor and in active labor
    a. Principles, objectives, and expectations
    b. Support during *early* labor and *active* labor
      (1) Emotional and physical support
      (2) Setting up for an optimal transaction
      (3) Admission procedures
      (4) Comfort measures
    c. Breathing techniques
      (1) Principles
      (2) Demonstration and practice
    d. Positions for labor
  3. Support of the couple during transition, delivery, and early postpartum period
    a. Principles, objectives, and expectations
    b. Elements of support
      (1) Emotional and physical support
      (2) Procedures
      (3) Expectations of prepared couples
    c. Breathing techniques
      (1) Principles
      (2) Demonstration and practice
    d. Positions for birth
    e. Parental attachment
  4. Support of the couple during special situations and procedures
    a. Principles, objectives, and expectations
    b. Special situations and procedures
      (1) Induction and augmentation
      (2) Monitoring
      (3) Prolonged first stage
      (4) Prolonged second stage
      (5) Use of medication
      (6) Cesarean births
    c. Nursing intervention and techniques

Although material presented in this brief outline deals mainly with knowledge acquisition, the underlying philosophy of the curriculum must be one of attitudinal change. It is vital to present all new information within the framework of a family-centered philosophy, emphasizing both the staff's and the family's rights and responsibilities.

GROUP PROCESS

While theoretic content and skills are being upgraded, it is important to deal with staff feelings on an ongoing basis. As discussed in the previous chapter, for change. It is vital to present all new information within the framework of a family-cognitive material is presented and staff attitudes are ignored, change will not happen.

Staff meetings to discuss feelings are vital. The first meeting could use an attitudinal survey about family-centered maternity care to begin discussion. There is an example of such a survey below.

The leader for these staff meetings must be nonjudgmental and willing and able to discuss all issues related to family-centered maternity care. Discussion should include advantages and disadvantages of proposed changes, in addition to staff feelings. During these meetings it may be helpful to present examples of hospital maternity units in which family-centered maternity care is a reality.

As nursing staff members try out their new, expanded roles, a "buddy system" may be helpful. Assigning a labor and delivery nurse to a newborn nursery with an experienced nursery nurse as preceptor can help ease the first few days in the new role. Also, positive reinforcement from all involved is vital as each nurse progresses. And, of course, since medical staff paraprofessionals and all auxiliary personnel are included in this challenging new provision of care, in-service classes and discussion groups must be designed for each level.

When developing family-centered maternity care, it is essential for staff nurses to accept the importance of continuous support for the laboring family and that such support may involve crossing 8-hour duty shifts. Acceptance of these basic premises helps staff nurses realize that they are not being replaced. Instead, they are part of a team whose goal is to help provide a quality birth experience under optimum conditions.

Family-centered maternity care survey

Please complete the following phrases in your own words. Do not take time to think through and analyze your response. Simply react. It is not necessary to sign this paper or to identify yourself in any way. When each person has finished writing, we will exchange papers and have a discussion.

Family-centered maternity care is _____

Mothers and babies _____

Mothers need _____

Fathers need _____

Babies need _____

Siblings need _____

Breastfeeding is _____

Bonding is _____

Fathers' presence at birth is _____

Assigning nurses to care for mother/baby units is _____
_____

Right now I feel _____

A critical element in the implementation of the Manchester program was provided by the first monitrice who served as a nonthreatening role model for the staff nurses. Formerly a staff nurse in pediatrics, this monitrice was nonetheless an outsider in the labor and delivery unit. But the staff nurses perceived the family's enthusiasm and happy results from the very beginning. The advantages of continuous support, both psychologically and physiologically, were obvious immediately. In addition, the rewards in terms of personal satisfaction for the monitrice were obvious. Deep interpersonal bonds established between the laboring family and monitrice provided fulfillment and feelings of accomplishment. This exemplified in a very real way the highest calling of the nursing professional—the art of caring.

An additional benefit was that staff nurses were motivated to provide two classes in prepared childbirth in the hospital. Since these classes were subsidized by staff obstetricians, they were free to expectant couples.

PARENTING EDUCATION

Classes in preparation for the birth itself are only a small part of an extensive preparation for parenthood program that should be available to all childbearing people, whether single or in couples. Such a program recognizes that pregnancy is not a disease, but a state of wellness during which people move from the role of expectant parents to the role and responsibilities of parents of a new baby, as a new family. Pregnancy can be a meaningful growth experience and can increase the family's self-confidence with the help of education for parenting.

A typical preparation for parenthood program recognizes that childbearing people have different interests and informational needs as the pregnancy progresses; consequently the program is designed to meet the concerns of the people at the three major stages of pregnancy and after birth.

Early pregnancy ("early bird") classes provide fundamental information about early development, understanding physiologic and emotional changes of pregnancy, human sexuality, and the nutritional needs of the mother and fetus.

Midpregnancy classes provide information on preparation for breast and bottle feeding, basic hygiene, health maintenance (rest, exercise, nutrition), and infant health.

Late pregnancy (preparation for childbirth) classes discuss support systems for pregnancy and after delivery, so families can function independently and effectively by developing their own health awareness and maintenance behavior.

After birth classes ("what do we do now?") cover coping mechanisms for the reality of parenting, support systems, infant care, growth, and development, birth control methods, human sexuality and adapting to new roles (wife/lover/mother and husband/lover/father).

During all the classes, open expression of feelings and concerns about any aspect of pregnancy, birth, or parenting is welcomed.

It is important to recognize that preparation for labor began as a consumer movement, and for a long time many of the classes were developed largely by consumers. The movement immigrated here from Europe, first through the pioneering efforts of Grantly Dick-Read from England, whose book *Childbirth Without Fear* planted the seed. After World War II prepared childbirth gained momentum through the popularization of the Lamaze method by authors such as Dr. Lamaze *(Painless Childbirth)*, Marjorie Karmel *(Thank You Dr. Lamaze)*, and Elisabeth Bing *(Six Practical Lessons for an Easier Childbirth)*. The American Society for Psychoprophylaxis in Obstetrics (ASPO) was founded in 1960 to promote the philosophy and principles of the Lamaze method, and, thanks to the determined efforts of this organization and its many chapters and affiliates throughout the country, several thousand certified Lamaze childbirth educators are now helping tens of thousands of expectant couples enjoy the experience of birth through the Lamaze method. The ASPO, through its strict adherence to the fundamental principles of psychoprophylaxis, has been primarily responsible for the creation of a new professional—the childbirth educator.

Because professional childbirth educators have diverse backgrounds, they have brought a richness and diversity to this new profession that could not have been obtained if it were limited to nurses alone.

SUMMARY

When planning to provide family-centered care, it is important to remember that nurses make up the largest group of health care professionals in this country and are responsible for much of the care given to childbearing families. The potential that nurses have for influencing change in maternity care is unlimited. However, in assuming the role of childbirth educator, nurses need to be aware that individualized care of the childbearing family implies options and that no single group has all the answers. Many persons and many disciplines have the potential to make significant contributions to the total birth experience.

Family-centered nursing does make a difference. It has the potential to change attitudes about birth and parenting for the better. The time has come for nurses to actively support the family in childbearing and parenting as *normal experiences*.

REFERENCES

1. Aiken, L. H.: Primary care: the challenge for nursing, Am. J. Nurs. **77**(11):1828-1832, 1977.
2. Aspy, V. H., and Roebuck, F. N.: Considering patient-centered obstetric nursing care: why and how?, JOGN Nurs. **8**(5):297-301, 1979.
3. Brown, M. S., and Hurlock, J. T.: Mothering the mother, Am. J. Nurs. **77**(3):438-441, 1977.
4. Ciske, K. L.: Accountability—the essence of primary nursing, Am. J. Nurs. **79**(5):890-894, 1979.

5. Dahlen, A. L.: With primary nursing we have it all together, Am. J. Nurs. **78**(3):426-428, 1978.

6. Doering, S. G., and Entwisle, D. R.: Preparation during pregnancy and ability to cope with labor and delivery, Am. J. Orthopsychiatry **45**:825-837, 1975.

7. Freeman, M. H.: Giving family life a good start in the hospital, Am. J. MCN **4**(1):51-54, 1979.

8. Henneborn, W. J., and Cogan, R.: The effect of husband participation on reported pain and probability of medication during labor and birth J. Psychosom. Res. **19**:215-222, 1975.

9. Hommel, F.: Nurses in private practice as monitrices, Am. J. Nurs. **69**:1447-1450, 1969.

10. Kowalski, K. E.: "On call" staffing, Am. J. Nurs. **73**:1725-1727, 1973.

11. Lamaze, F.: Painless childbirth, psychoprophylactic method, Chicago, 1958, Henry Regnery Co.

12. Manchester Monitrice Associates: The birth of a monitrice, Manchester, Conn., 1977.

13. Norr, K. L., Block, C. R., Charles, A., et al.: Explaining pain and enjoyment in childbirth, J. Health Soc. Behav. pp. 260-275, 1977.

14. Read, G. D.: Childbirth without fear, New York, 1944, Harper & Bros.

CHAPTER 6

Questions and answers

This chapter contains questions and answers by Philip Sumner about some common concerns about birthing rooms and birthing programs.

1. Are elective inductions a part of your practice?

Because of the risks of elective induction—iatrogenic prematurity, fetal distress due to anoxia, prolapsed cord, premature separation of the placenta, and malpresentation—we limit our inductions to those which are indicated medically. However, in labors where there is no progress and weak contractions, there may be a need for oxytocin (Pitocin) stimulation. We believe Nature knows best and prefer to await the onset of spontaneous labor whenever possible.

Maisels and co-workers[18] forced a refocus on the issue of elective delivery (induction). Elective delivery was defined as one in which there is no medical condition of the mother or fetus that could be interpreted as indicating the necessity for immediate delivery.

In their study,[18] 38 infants (almost 4% of admissions) were admitted to the regional neonatal center, following elective induction, from 20 hospitals in the referral area. Of these babies, 87% were delivered by cesarean birth. These facts are disturbing for at least two reasons. First, it is probable that not every affected neonate was transferred to the center. In other words, the scope of the problem exceeds 4%. For example, Goldenberg and Nelson[10] concluded that at least 15% and possibly 33% of their cases of hyaline membrane disease (HMD) resulted from inappropriate obstetric management. Second, these cases are now preventable by fetal maturity assessment *or* by awaiting labor.

Eighteen of the neonates[18] developed HMD (6.4% of HMD admissions). One newborn died. The cost of total care amounted to $62,201 (median $2678). Conservative estimates place the cost at an annual national figure exceeding $16 million. The expenditure of monies and life in elective deliveries not associated with assured fetal maturity is becoming increasingly more difficult to justify.

2. Would you please comment on the increasing cesarean birthrate in the United States and the comparatively low cesarean rate in your program?

First, I am so pleased that you used the term cesarean birth instead of cesarean section. Terminology is very important when communicating with childbearing families. The word "section" carries with it a surgical connotation and minimizes the "birth" aspect of the experience.[7]

The cesarean birthrate has been rising 2% per year nationally, and in some hospitals it has reached an astronomic figure of over 40%. I believe the present high-risk childbirth model is creating more anxiety than obstetric personnel can handle, and the increasing cesarean rate is in part a manifestation of this anxiety. Maternity staffs need to treat their own anxiety, as well as that of the mother, by creating a more reassuring environment in which all can relax and allow Mother Nature a chance.

There are valid explanations for an increase in the cesarean birthrate. These include better nutrition with less emphasis on weight gain limitations, larger babies, older mothers, lower parity, and births by second and third generation women who were themselves born by cesarean methods because of cephalopelvic disproportion. The cesarean rate is always higher for nulliparas compared with multiparas. In fact, in our hospital it is three times as great. With an ever increasing percentage of births being to nulliparous women, a rise in the cesarean rate is inevitable. In our practice 15 years ago 20% of mothers were having first babies and 80% at least their second. During 1979 58% of our mothers were having their first baby. This represents a tripling of the percentage of nulliparas, which means that one might expect a tripling of the cesarean rate.

Other factors, such as elective inductions, intravenous oxytocin (Pitocin) stimulation of labor, electronic fetal monitoring, artificial rupture of membranes, and medications and anesthesia when used inappropriately, may under certain circumstances contribute to the rise in cesarean births.[15] These reasons may be more difficult to justify.

Although some women who have had cesarean deliveries may be able to have subsequent vaginal births, most need repeat cesarean delivery, perpetuating the concept of birth as a surgical procedure. The costs of such surgical procedures are high in terms of dollars spent as well as maternal morbidity. Preoccupation with the condition of the fetus often overshadows concern for maternal well-being and the long-term implications for the family. Although the proponents of cesarean births often emphasize their goal of reducing perinatal morbidity, they should also consider the potentially excessive maternal morbidity and mortality associated with this procedure.

Evrard and Golch[8] reviewed data from all births in Rhode Island from 1965 to

1975. During this period the rate of cesarean births rose from 6.41% to 14.07%. There were 162,656 deliveries and 20 deaths directly related to obstetric problems. Seven of these deaths were associated with other procedures or with abnormal pregnancies. Of the remaining 13, a "disproportionate number" were linked to cesarean deliveries, a rate of 6.95 per 10,000; there were four deaths among 149,715 vaginal deliveries, a rate of 0.27 per 10,000. Comparison of these rates shows "a risk factor 26 times greater for cesarean section than for vaginal deliveries." Because of the excessive maternal mortality involved, the researchers analyzed the nine cesarean-related deaths more closely.

> The indications for the sections were straightforward: abruptio placentae (2) cephalopelvic disproportion (1), repeat cesarean section (3), preeclampsia (1), placenta previa (1), transverse lie (1). The complications eventuating in the deaths were ultimately ascribable to sepsis (7), hemorrhage (1), and anesthesia complications.

This analysis reaffirms a "crucial question," according to Evrard and Golch[8]: "Is the risk of death inherent in the cesarean section per se, or is it more likely due to the associated obstetric complication for which the cesarean section was performed?" In their view, the *procedure itself* was responsible for four of the nine deaths: the three repeat cesarean sections and an abruptio placentae after 10 hours of labor with intact membranes.

"While it may be argued," they[8] continue, "that by adopting the newer and expanded indications for cesarean section there will be a decrease in traumatic vaginal delivery with consequent improved outcome for the fetus and possibly for the parturient, the absolute increase in primary cesarean sections may result in higher maternal morbidity and mortality."

Of course, not to be overlooked or underemphasized are the psychologic aspects of cesarean birth—particularly for the woman who undergoes an unexpected cesarean. These women frequently feel gypped, realizing that they may never be able to experience a "natural" vaginal delivery. These women and their families have unique needs, requiring especially supportive medical and nursing care.[19]

I believe one of our greatest needs is to develop and improve techniques for vaginal delivery for obstetric problems, rather than resort to the cesarean as the panacea. For example, ambulation and creative positioning of the woman in labor may be very useful. It is possible that rocking and circular rotation of the pelvis may aid internal rotation and descent of the fetal head. The joints are softened at term. By the mother slowly rotating the pelvis during pushing contractions, the point of maximum pressure for the descending fetal head is constantly in motion. This is similar to the twisting motion one exerts on a cork to replace it in a bottle, and I have found it to be a very useful technique in many instances.

3. Is electronic fetal monitoring used routinely in the birth room?

Although I am not opposed in principle to the concept of continuous surveillance of the fetal heart, I believe, along with many others, that the science of fetal monitoring is still in its infancy. Although its routine use appears to have a valid place in the management of high-risk labors, it should be used selectively in normal labors. It is not its use but its depersonalizing effect that concerns me. We should first give constant human surveillance with the "fetal monitrice" a chance and acknowledge that the well-trained human ear is capable of recognizing bradycardia, tachycardia, and the quality of the fetal heart. We *must* not automatically upgrade technology and downgrade the human element.

Electronic fetal monitoring is used in the birth rooms if our "fetal monitrice" feels that she needs the additional data it could provide. This decision is based on her careful and continuous assessment of the laboring woman and her fetus. Also, in the event that intravenous oxytocin (Pitocin) is needed for augmentation or the rare induction of labor, electronic fetal monitoring is useful because of increased risk to the fetus. I feel that using the electronic monitor as an assessment tool *when indicated* is totally within the scope of safe obstetrics for the 1980s. However, not infrequently the fetal monitor may draw some "nonreassuring" or "ominous" patterns on the graph, and suddenly a physiologic situation is converted into a potentially pathologic one. We anticipate trouble, our anxiety level rises, our confidence wanes, and the decision to deliver the baby abdominally is made. Had the woman been managed in a more relaxed and physiologic manner, in a more supportive environment, the nonreassuring pattern either might not have occurred or might have reverted to a reassuring pattern in time for her to have a normal vaginal delivery.

Battaglia and Hellegers,[5] after conducting extensive in-depth discussions with individuals concerned with the well-being of the fetus and newborn, have concluded as follows:

> The use of continuous fetal monitoring, scalp vein analysis, and amnioscopy represent techniques of intense supervision of patients. Whether the good results obtainable with these techniques are due to close supervision of patients is not clear. No practitioner can, with the present state of the art, be considered negligent for not performing these three tests. He can be considered negligent for not supervising his patients. Until such time as adequately designed studies establish the full validity of the tests themselves, they should not be considered a replacement for clinical judgment but only an adjunct to it.

In 1976, Albert Haverkamp[12] wrote a definitive article on fetal monitoring in high-risk pregnancy, stating, "Although monitoring is a helpful adjunct in observing labor, other ways, including auscultation (listening to the fetal heart with a fetoscope), may turn out to be adequate, especially in smaller hospitals where procurement and proper use of sophisticated monitoring equipment may not be feasible." In another study, reported in 1979, Haverkamp[11] randomly assigned 690 high-risk mothers to one of three monitoring groups: auscultation, electronic fetal monitoring alone, or electronic fetal monitoring with the option of scalp sampling. There were no differences between monitored and control groups in immediate infant outcomes. In the electronically monitored groups, the cesarean birthrate was markedly increased (18%) as compared with the auscultated group (6%).

These studies suggest that monitoring of normal laboring women by auscultation according to the protocol of Haverkamp and colleagues[12] may suffice. Haverkamp's protocol includes recording fetal heart rate (FHR) every 15 minutes in first stage and every 5 minutes in second stage.

Harold Schulman,[25] Chairman of the Department of Obstetrics/Gynecology at Albert Einstein College, wrote a paper in which he stated that there was an absence of good correlation between abnormal FHR patterns and neonatal conditions: "We have been unable to demonstrate an ideological rationale between various fetal heart rate patterns and clinical entities."

Banta and Thacker[4] conducted a careful review of the literature on benefits, risks, and costs of electronic fetal monitoring. Their review disclosed little, if any, increased benefit from electronic fetal monitoring compared with auscultation, except in the instance of low birthweight infants.

A National Institute of Health task force[20] has formally stated that periodic auscultation of the FHR is an acceptable method of monitoring the low-risk fetus. The task force[27] also said that "the medical record should reflect careful consideration of the benefits and risks to each individual, including a discussion of the indications for electronic fetal monitoring with the patient."

In summary, since its introduction in 1960 electronic fetal monitoring has increased in use until it is estimated that today it is used in over 50% of labors in the United States.[14] Review of the literature on fetal monitoring discloses numerous studies that present data both for and against its use. Many more investigations are needed before the growing controversy about fetal monitoring can be resolved. In the meantime, however, we will continue to upgrade the human support during labor by depending on our "fetal monitrices," whose presence has so many subtle favorable effects on the course of labor.

4. Would you comment on the Leboyer method of birth?

Dr. Leboyer's[17] great contribution has been his insistence that the newborn infant is to be respected as a human being who can react violently and permanently to a hospital birth, which he says can be traumatic. Leboyer, author of *Birth Without Violence,* suggested radical departures from traditional hospital maternity practices. Leboyer delivered babies into an environment that is kept warm, quiet, and softly lit—unlike the usual delivery room with its bright light, cool temperature,

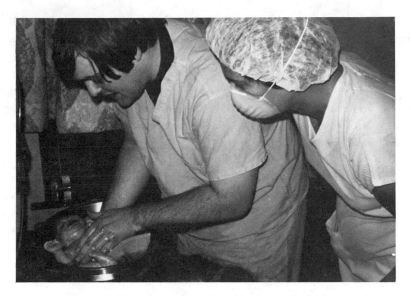

Fig. 6-1. A Leboyer bath in the birth room.

and sounds presumably strange and harsh to the newborn. The births I witnessed in the Lamaze Clinic in 1967 with Dr. Vellay were as sensitively handled as anything that Dr. Leboyer described. The difference is that Dr. Vellay has emphasized the total experience of mother, father, and baby, whereas Dr. Leboyer has concentrated almost exclusively on the infant's reactions and sensitivity during and immediately after birth.

In the Leboyer[17] method, the physician delivers the baby gently, bringing him out of the birth canal slowly, and placing him on the mother's bare abdomen

The procedures last for about 12 minutes altogether, but Leboyer and his supporters maintain the benefits are life-long, since the initial imprinting on the baby's consciousness and emotions is profound.

An interesting study[21] done to examine the effects of the Leboyer method of delivery illustrates the importance of the gentleness of delivery rather than use of a specific method. In this study 28 mothers were assigned to a Leboyer group and 26 to a control group for a gentle, but conventional delivery. There were no significant differences noted in maternal or newborn morbidity or in infant behavior at either 24 or 72 hours post partum. The investigators concluded that their results failed to show statistically significant advantages to a Leboyer delivery. Since both study groups were treated with principles of gentleness, the results suggest that gentle conventional deliveries can indeed produce outcomes similar to those of Leboyer deliveries.

The immersion of a newborn in warm water, suctioning, or the use of gloves is secondary to the concept of extreme patience and sensitivity that predominates in Leboyer's method. He is simply concerned with developing a sensitivity to the family's needs.[23] Too much emphasis has been placed on the warm bath given to the baby by the father immediately after birth. Although such a bath is available in the birthing room if the parents insist, we prefer the expression, "bathe the baby in parental love" through the many tender and meaningful interactions between parents and newborn.

5. Do you have provision for home follow-up of families after hospital discharge?

Our nurse practitioners have a policy of telephoning postpartum mothers if they or their babies have had a complication of any kind. In addition, the Lamaze instructor phones the family at home and checks on them. If there is a serious problem identified, or if the family has elected the early discharge program (12 hours post partum), a visiting nurse will make home visits.

Also, in our community there is a consumer group of parents interested in improving the quality of childbirth and parenting. This FOCIS group (Family Oriented Childbirth Information Society) offers classes during both prenatal and postpartum periods. Their emphasis post partum is on adjustment to parenting. FOCIS is really an outgrowth of the family-centered program in which couples accept responsibility for their lives. The total medical services available to a family giving birth is far more than the hospital alone can offer; it comes from active involvement of the community itself in the birth process.

6. Do birth rooms conflict with state and federal health regulations?

Being the first hospital in Connecticut to establish this type of program, there was no model to follow or special regulations to adhere to. Once arrangements were made through the hospital administration to obtain the appropriate equipment and nursing coverage, we began using our first birth room without consulting the state or federal government before hand. As the program developed, there were periodic inspections made by state authorities. They have been supportive of our program, asking no probing or unusual questions and applying the same standards to birth rooms as to regular delivery rooms.

7. What do you see as the potential effects on normal childbirth of consolidation of perinatal care?

I feel that the trend toward consolidation of obstetric units into large, impersonal places far from the homes of both the woman and her physician is not conducive to participatory childbirth and poses a potential threat to the community hospital, which should remain the primary birth facility. In a larger center, the mother is more likely to be managed using the high-risk, technologic model, whether she needs it or not. Once consolidation is accomplished the obstetrician will, in all probability, take gynecologic practice to the regional hospital, placing the pediatrician under increased pressure to admit children and adolescents there also, since the newborns are there. Suddenly, the local hospital's broad services to the community are threatened, and its future effectiveness may be placed in jeopardy. Since the majority of expectant mothers are healthy, it would make more sense to have them give birth in the community hospital. Even many high-risk mothers can have deliveries in the community hospital, provided appropriate consultation is available. Transfer is, in itself, traumatic and should be kept to a minimum.

A further problem with obstetric consolidation is the tendency to treat every pregnancy as high risk, in need of all the management of the most delicate and dangerous surgical procedures. This often prevents Nature from doing what it is best equipped to do. Many of these centers are so oriented to medical and surgical intervention that they are graduating residents who have seldom seen a completely "natural" birth. For the relatively small percentage of pregnant women who require the expertise of the university center, I have no hesitation recommending that they go there. In this sense, consolidation of obstetric services is indeed a constructive step forward. However, such high-risk pregnancies can usually be screened early on and are the exception, not the rule. Each mother is an individual, and the degree of risk is a continuum.

8. Would you consider working with certified nurse-midwives in birth rooms?

Yes, I would. I feel that competent midwives can manage normal births and call on the obstetrician for the complicated ones. Most nurse-midwives have great skill and patience and can dedicate more time to the childbearing family, since they do not have to do gynecologic surgery. I can envision a time when our specialty will not focus solely on the birth itself but rather on mother, infant, and father during the crucial, formative years. In such a simple, joyous, yet medically sound model for childbirth the certified nurse-midwife is an important member of the team. In fact, I feel that the efforts of the growing number of certified nurse-midwives have contributed significantly to the rise of the alternative birth movement. In many alternative birth centers throughout the United States the midwife is the primary caregiver.

Gatewood and Stewart[9] of Americus, Georgia, have reported about their team approach in private practice. In the first year that they incorporated two nurse-midwives into their practice, these midwives presided at the births of 61% of the vaginally delivered babies. The childbearing women, nurse-midwives, and obstetricians were all pleased with the team approach.

In our practice we have found nurse practitioners to be an invaluable contribution to prenatal and postpartum care. All prenatal women are seen by nurse practitioners, as well as all three obstetricians.

9. How do you feel about home births?

Although I am happy to work with midwives and feel that there is a great and beneficial use for midwifery, I believe that the need for them is best fulfilled within the hospital. Home deliveries, whether under the guidance of a midwife or physician, present unnecessary hazard to mother and infant, especially since we do not have the services of mobile emergency squads. Even though many obstetricians do not support the home birth movement, I believe that many of us can sympathize with it as a reaction to our specialty's insensitivity to the needs of the modern woman. There are choices to be made, and the mother demands the right to share in the decisions. If we do not sanction home birth, we must equally discourage routine and unnecessary intervention. Yet, when complications develop, the "expert" opinion is often that more gadgets should have been used and intervention started earlier. This not only confuses the woman who wants to and can manage her own labor, but it also forces the obstetrician who wants to work along with her into practicing defensive medicine.

10. What do you mean by a "modified" paracervical block, and what is the instance of fetal bradycardia following use of this technique?

No anesthetic or anesthetic technique is without the risk of side effects.

Although I realize that routine paracervical blocks have caused some controversy, in our 17 years of experience with modified paracervical blocks adverse side effects for both mother and baby have been extremely rare. We have found a modified paracervical block to be a relatively simple procedure, effectively blocking both the sympathetic and parasympathetic afferent nerve pathways.

No special vaginal preparation is necessary. The mother is positioned slightly diagonal in bed, with legs in a "frog" position to provide easy access to injection sites.

An Iowa trumpet guide and 10-ml Luer-Lok syringe are the only pieces of equipment needed. The two purposes of the Iowa trumpet guide are (1) to allow accurate placement of the needle in the lateral vaginal vault and (2) to prevent excessive depth of penetration. When inserting the needle into the guide, it is important that only the bevel of the needle protrudes from the guide by positioning the malleable bead near the hub of the needle in such a way that excessive penetration is impossible.

A 10-ml Luer-Lok syringe is loaded with appropriate anesthetic. A needle is attached to this syringe and placed on a sterile tray. The Iowa trumpet guide is

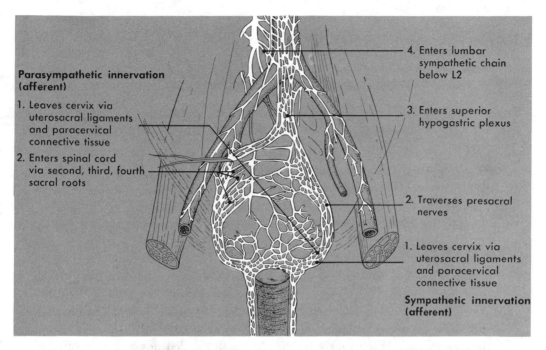

Parasympathetic innervation (afferent)

1. Leaves cervix via uterosacral ligaments and paracervical connective tissue

2. Enters spinal cord via second, third, fourth sacral roots

4. Enters lumbar sympathetic chain below L2

3. Enters superior hypogastric plexus

2. Traverses presacral nerves

1. Leaves cervix via uterosacral ligaments and paracervical connective tissue

Sympathetic innervation (afferent)

Fig. 6-2. Parasympathetic and sympathetic innervation (afferent)—anteroposterior view.

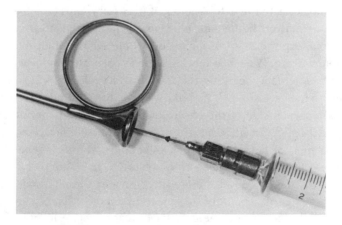

Fig. 6-3. Needle partially inserted into Iowa trumpet needle guide; note lead bead.

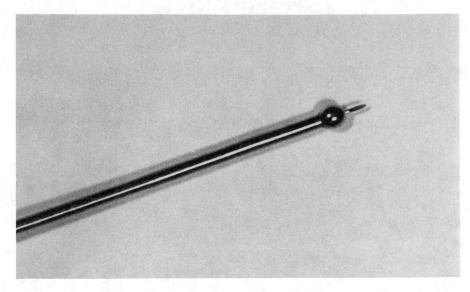

Fig. 6-4. Needle point extending a short distance beyond guide.

passed into the vaginal vault along the lateral aspect of the examiner's finger, which is lateral to the cervix. The predetermined placement of the bead will permit the tip of the needle to penetrate only submucosally (Fig. 6-4). Following aspiration the anesthetic is injected submucosally, raising a weal.

The anesthetic may be slowly injected in small divided doses of mepivacaine 1% (Carbocaine) or other local anesthetic agents into the lateral vaginal vaults. Injection sites are at one or any combination of the following: 2, 3, 4, 8, 9, and 10 o'clock, *well lateral* to the cervix, depending on location of discomfort (Fig. 6-5). The block may be repeated in 1 to 2 hours, if necessary.

This procedure has an immediate effect with minimal side effects or systemic absorption. In our experience at Manchester Memorial Hospital, fetal bradycardia has been extremely rare. A clinical investigation is currently under way that should provide more specific data regarding the use of paracervical blocks in our practice.

The original paracervical block techniques usually required injections of 10 ml of lidocaine 1% on each side of the cervix, with the needle penetrating the fornix approximately 1.5 cm (³/₄ inch). Use of this technique does not take into consideration the importance of lateral superficial injections. There is general agreement that fetal response to a paracervical block is related to the dosage of local anesthetic administered. Also, the spread of the anesthetic agent through maternal tissues is probably related to the placement of the injecting needle. Consequently, by reducing the dosage of the anesthetic agent to its lowest effective level and injecting it shallowly, well lateral under the mucosa, fetal bradycardia is extremely rare.

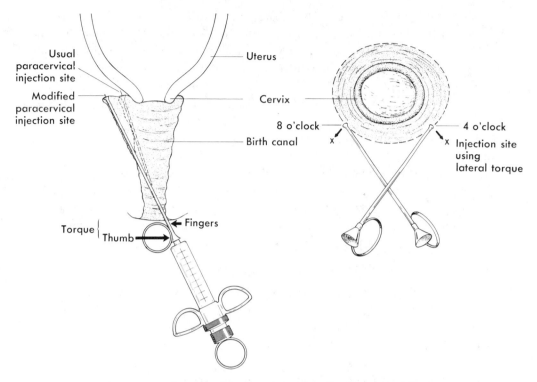

Fig. 6-5. Usual and modified injection sites for paracervical block.

It is important to stress that we use paracervical block anesthesia only for laboring women who need it and then only in small amounts intended to reduce discomfort to tolerable levels, but not necessarily eliminate it. In keeping with our philosophy of nonintervention, it would be ideal if we never had to use any medication for pain relief in labor. Since every kind of medication used in childbirth poses some risk to the mother, the baby, or both,[2] our goal is always to *minimize* the amount of medication required and never to use analgesic drugs or paracervical blocks routinely. Optimum individual care implies choices for clinicians as well as consumers. We believe that the modified paracervical block is one of the most valuable techniques to enable us to achieve the goals of the prepared childbirth era, although other anesthetic techniques are compatible with these goals as well.

11. What is the average length of time couples stay in the hospital after birth?

Couples usually remain in the hospital for 48 to 72 hours after their birth experiences. Although they are free to go home at any time in the postpartum period, we do encourage new families to remain in the hospital at least 12 hours.

Our hospital has the policy of not charging the patient for the day of discharge. For example, if a mother was admitted to the hospital on a Monday morning and then delivered her baby that afternoon, she would be encouraged to remain until after physicians' rounds at approximately 10 A.M. the following morning. There would be no charge for that Tuesday morning in the hospital.

Our 12-hour postpartum early discharge policy is used by less than 10% of our childbearing population. When people elect to follow the early discharge plan, there must be no maternal or infant complications requiring nursing or medical management.

In keeping with our philosophy of individualizing care, we first assess the family's support system at home. If all involved agree that it would be helpful, we make arrangements for visiting nurse follow-up, even for those who go home on the second or third postpartum day. Such follow-up consists of at least one daily visit for a minimum of 4 postpartum days.

12. Are birthing rooms expensive to build and operate?

Not at all. Any existing labor room that has dimensions of 9 by 12 feet can be converted into a birthing room. The expenses involved in initial alterations will depend on how much conversion must be done to achieve a safe delivery setting. Wall suction and oxygen will be needed. Other amenities include wallpaper, drapes on windows or false windows if none exist, pictures, telephone, storage cabinets, and a radio for music. Medical equipment needed is already owned by hospitals and will simply have to be stored out of sight when possible.

Of course, the most important piece of equipment in the birth room is a labor-delivery bed. These beds range in price from $2000 to $8000. Once this initial investment is made, only maintenance costs are involved. Actually, it has been our experience that birthing rooms are less expensive to operate than traditional delivery rooms because they conserve space, staff, linen, and supplies.

In 1975 Esther Adkins[1] reported on savings realized in the all-in-one unit for birth at Bronson Methodist Hospital in Kalamazoo, Michigan. She emphasized the considerable savings that can be realized in linen, equipment usage, and personnel time. In fact, Adkins proposed that savings in linen usage and personnel time in the unit described could be estimated at $1000 per year. In addition, housekeeping time was decreased an estimated 21 minutes per delivery, which translates into a savings of approximately $3200 per year, according to 1975 costs.

13. What is the average rectal temperature of babies while in the birth rooms and on admission to the nursery?

The average rectal temperature of babies in the newborn nursery between 30 minutes and 1 hour after birth is 97.7° F. Remember, all babies are dried quickly and placed next to their mother's warm body. A hat made from stockinette is placed on the baby's head to prevent heat loss. Also, a radiant heat panel is used in the birth room as a source of additional overhead heat for the new family. Ambient air temperature in the room is kept at 70° to 72° F.

An infant loses body heat by (1) evaporation, (2) radiation, (3) convection, and (4) conduction.[24]

Evaporative heat loss occurs when moisture evaporates from wet skin in a relatively dry atmosphere. A baby wet with amniotic fluid in an air-conditioned delivery room rapidly loses a great deal of body heat this way. Evaporative heat loss can be minimized by drying the baby thoroughly immediately after birth.

Loss by radiation results when heat transfers from the body surface to cooler surfaces of surrounding objects, e.g., incubator wall, room wall, and windows cooled by air-conditioners. Loss by radiation is minimized by wrapping or covering the dry baby with a warm blanket.

Convective heat loss is increased by surrounding air currents, cold oxygen, and cold air blown by air-conditioners. Heat is also lost by *conduction* to cooler objects in direct contact with the baby's skin, e.g., diapers, blankets, scales, instruments, and hands.[24] Convective heat loss can be prevented by protecting the baby from cold drafts and keeping the birth room warm.

In 1974 a study[24] of 115 infants compared temperatures of those placed in heated beds with those held by their mothers on the delivery table. The difference between the mean temperatures of the two groups was not significant. Subsequent studies[6,13] have confirmed these findings, indicating that removing the normal newborn from his mother and placing him in a heated bed to keep warm is not necessary. An optimum heat-conserving situation exists with direct skin-to-skin contact between parent and infant.

14. What type of apparel does the hospital staff wear in birthing rooms?

Staff members wear the same type of apparel that they wear in a standard delivery room. Since the mother and father share the same constellation of bacteria, the father is not required to wear a cap or mask, but hospital scrub clothes are still worn.

15. Will insurance companies provide reimbursement for monitrice services?

The answer is a qualified yes. Actually, it depends on the insurance company involved. This has been a sore point for which we have sought a solution for several years. Insurance companies are now beginning to realize that the monitrice provides an essential support service, like a private duty nurse, often eliminating the need for an anesthesiologist. The reduced need for anesthesia improves the outcome of the birth experience for mother and baby and shortens the hospital stay. The result for the insurance company is reduced cost, and therefore more and more are recognizing the validity of the monitrice concept.

16. Will insurance companies provide reimbursement for births in birth rooms?

Insurance companies make no differentiation whatsoever in the amount of compensation for births in regular delivery rooms and births in birth rooms. The charge at Manchester Memorial for using birth rooms is $25 less than that for delivery room use because of the economy of nursing services and equipment needed in birth rooms.

17. Have your malpractice insurance premiums increased since your practice incorporated birthing rooms?

No, for insurance purposes there is no differentiation between births that occur in a standard delivery room and those in a birth room. Malpractice insurance policies do not recognize use of birth rooms as creating a greater probability of malpractice claims. In fact, we feel that since the birthing room program helps to humanize birth, we are creating a less anxiety-producing atmosphere. Such an atmosphere may well be less likely to produce a lawsuit, even if we should encounter major problems with either the mother or baby.

18. How is sibling visitation implemented after birth?

A comfortable sibling visitation room has been established in the hospital adjacent to our maternity unit. When the mother returns to her postpartum room, she is given the sibling visitation book so that she may reserve the room for any $^1/_2$ hour available each day, or a second $^1/_2$ hour, if available.

We limit use of the room to one family at a time. The newborn is brought into the sibling room so that the entire family may visit together. Studies have documented the importance of sibling visitation and the positive effect that short visits to their mother can have on children's behavior.[26] Other hospitals include siblings at birth, also, but this sibling visiting room for after-birth family visits has worked very well for us. Several small, short-term studies[3,22] present encouraging findings concerning siblings at birth. However, we are not sure of the long-term effect of presence at the birth itself on preschool children. I am skeptical about including small children at birth until we have longitudinal studies to review.

19. How will birthing rooms and a program such as yours benefit the hospital?

The hospital will, of course, benefit medically but also in nonmedical ways. First of all, with large community acceptance and enthusiasm, the hospital's image is changed. Instead of being thought of as an impenetrable fortress, the community hospital is seen as a progressive, humanized institution and a focus for family and community education. Ultimately, through this improved image, the volume of births in the hospital will increase. In addition, consumers satisfied with childbirth there will return when their families need general medical care. The benefits are indeed long term.

20. In your program are all women routinely shaved prior to delivery?

We have eliminated all *routine* perineal shavings, enemas, intravenous infusions, etc. Since our program individualizes care, we determine each family's needs separately. Because an episiotomy may be necessary, a single midline shaving of the perineal area is all that is done. Studies[16] show that shaving does not improve the sterilization of the perineal skin, so if there is any shaving done, it is merely to improve visualization of the area for episiotomy repair.

21. How have leaders in perinatal care responded to your program?

We have received numerous enthusiastic responses from all areas of the United States and from countries around the world. Typical examples follow.

> We noted with great interest your recent article entitled "The Labor-Delivery Bed—Simplified Obstetrics," published in the Journal of Reproductive Medicine in October, 1974. There are some excellent points to your discussion and logic, and I feel that your good results are probably understated in that there is no way to properly measure the satisfaction and pleasure experienced by the patient and her husband. As you can note, we are in complete accord with your well-stated approach to the modern-day management of labor and delivery.*

> • • •

> Great, great, great! I am so glad to see your program. It bears out all of my convictions—that we can and must get on with a more joyous, less pathological model of childbirth. By reinforcing young parents' pathology (pregnancy as an illness, need for drugs, passivity, etc.) we are getting back what we should expect—one of two reactions: (1) more dependency and passivity than any of us can handle in our patients, including overuse of medication; or (2) revulsion and withdrawal from the system which labels them as damaged, or ill, or whatever. Either one is counterproductive for a young parent's self-image of him/herself as important to the new baby, but needing healthy support from a nurturing medical system. We've got to get on with it if we want to be in on a preventive model for early mother-father-infant interaction. Bravo to you and your group for your elegant efforts.†

> • • •

> John Kennell and I were most interested in the material you sent. Your very thoughtful reprint certainly described a most important experience with so many important elements that you have in your care—the continuous caring person, the preparation for childbirth, and all of the techniques that you worked out so nicely. You really are to be congratulated!‡

> • • •

> I was delighted to learn of your program and hope you continue to keep me informed. Your program is indeed rare, and for that reason it had not come to my attention before you wrote. I hope the success you have had will encourage more people to follow through on a more humanized approach to perinatal care.§

---

*Johnson, J.: Personal correspondence, 1975.
†Brazelton, T. B.: Personal correspondence, 1976.
‡Klaus, M. H.: Personal correspondence, 1976.
§Salk, L.: Personal correspondence, 1977.

REFERENCES

1. Adkins, E. L.: All-in-one unit improves patient care in OB, Hosp. Top. **53**(2):40-41, 1975.
2. American Academy of Pediatrics Committee on Drugs: Effect of medication during labor and delivery on infant outcome, Pediatrics **62**(3):402-403, 1978.
3. Anderson, S. V.: Siblings at birth: a survey and study, Birth and Family J. **6**(2):80-87, 1979.
4. Banta, D., and Thacker, S.: Electronic fetal monitoring: is it of benefit?, Birth and Family J. **6**(4):237-249, 1979.
5. Battaglia, F. C., and Hellegers, A. E.: Status of the fetus and newborn report of the Second Ross Conference on Obstetrical Research, Columbus, Ohio, 1973, Ross Labs.
6. Britton, G.: The effect of uninterrupted mother-infant contact post-delivery on two aspects of human maternal attachment and on temperature stabilization of the infant, unpublished masters thesis, University of Wisconsin, Madison, Wisc., 1977.
7. Donovan, B., and Allen, R. M.: The cesarean birth method, JOGN Nurs. **6**(6):37-48, 1977.
8. Evrard, J. R., et al.: Cesarean section and maternal mortality in Rhode Island, Obstet. Gynecol. **50**:594-597, Nov., 1977; as abstracted in Briefs, Jan., 1978, p. 3.
9. Gatewood, T. S., and Stewart, R. B.: Obstetricians and nurse-midwives: the team approach in private practice, Am. J. Obstet. Gynecol. **123**(1):35-40, 1975.
10. Goldenberg, R. L., et al.: Iatrogenic respiratory distress syndrome: an analysis of obstetric events preceding delivery of infants who develop respiratory distress syndrome, Am. J. Obstet. Gynecol. **123**:617-620, 1975.
11. Haverkamp, A., et al.: A controlled trial of the differential effects of intrapartum fetal monitoring, Am. J. Obstet. Gynecol. **134**(4):399-412, 1979.
12. Haverkamp, A., et al.: The evaluation of continuous heart rate monitoring in high-risk pregnancy, Am. J. Obstet. Gynecol. **12**(3):310-320, 1976.
13. Hill, S., and Shrank, L.: The effect of early parent-infant contact on newborn body temperature, JOGN Nurs. **8**(5):287-290, 1979.
14. Hobbins, J., Freeman, R., and Queens, J.: The fetal monitoring debate, Obstet. Gynecol. **54**(1):103-109, 1979.
15. Katz, B.: Unnatural childbirth, National Observer, Nov., 1976.
16. Landry, K. E., and Kilpatrick, D. M.: Why shave a mother before she gives birth?, Am. J. MCN **2**(3):189-190, 1977.
17. Leboyer, F.: Birth without violence, New York, 1975, Alfred A. Knopf.
18. Maisels, M. J., et al.: Elective delivery of the term fetus: an obstetrical hazard, J.A.M.A. **238**:2036, 1977.
19. Marut, J. S.: The special needs of the cesarean mother, Am. J. MCN **3**(4):202-206, 1978.
20. National Institutes of Health, and National Institute of Child and Human Development: Task force on predictors of fetal distress (draft), prepared as a working document for discussion at Consensus Development Conference on Antenatal Diagnosis, Bethesda, Md., NIH Publication No. 79-1973, April, 1979.
21. Nelson, N. M., et al.: A clinical trial of the Leboyer approach to childbirth, N. Engl. J. Med. **302**(12):655-660, 1980.
22. Perez, P.: Nuturing children who attend the birth of a sibling, Am. J. MCN **4**:215-217, 1979.
23. Phillips, C. R.: The essence of birth without violence, Am. J. MCN **1**(3):162-163, 1976.
24. Phillips, C. R.: Neonatal heat loss in heated cribs vs. mothers' arms, JOGN Nurs. **13**(6):11-14, 1974.
25. Schulman, H., et al.: Electronic fetal monitoring during labor, Obstet. Gynecol. **47**(6):706-710, 1976.
26. Trause, M. A.: Birth in the hospital: the effect on the sibling, Birth and Family J. **5**(4):207-210, 1978.
27. Zuspan, F. P., Quilligan, F. J., Iams, J. D., and vanGeign, H. P.: Predictors of intrapartum fetal distress: the role of electronic fetal monitoring, Am. J. Obstet. Gynecol. **135**(3):287-290, 1979.

CHAPTER 7

Other birth choices

For of all sad words of tongue or pen, the saddest are these: "It might have been."
John Greenleaf Whittier

In the past few years innovative alternatives to traditional birth have been springing up all over the United States. Some hospitals have simply modified their maternity services in an effort to humanize care. Others have instituted alternative birth centers, labor room birth policies, or birth rooms. Out-of-hospital birth centers have developed, offering hospital backup for emergencies. Following are descriptions from innovative health care providers about other birth choices within a hospital setting or in connection with a hospital.

ALTERNATIVE BIRTH CENTER, MOUNT ZION HOSPITAL AND MEDICAL CENTER, SAN FRANCISCO

The pioneering alternative birth center model developed at Mount Zion Hospital in San Francisco has had a great influence on the design of alternative birth centers in hospitals throughout the United States. The fundamental philosophic difference between the alternative birth center concept and a birthing room is screening criteria that divide the birthing population.

At Mount Zion, certified nurse-midwives have had hospital privileges since 1978. The staff designed criteria, policies, and procedures that have subsequently been used by many other hospital alternative birth centers. Some of this very thorough work follows.

STATEMENT OF PURPOSE

The provision of comprehensive perinatal services requires that the needs of low-risk as well as high-risk women and their infants be addressed. Concomitant with increasing sophistication in technical resources for management of high-risk obstetrical situations has come recognition on the part of providers that normal childbirth needs are not being met by traditional obstetrical practices. This recognition has been heightened by the advocacy position assumed by professional leaders, by childbirth educators, and by greater consumer participation in health care. The increased costs of traditional care have contributed to many young couples choosing home delivery, which offers the positive features of father and fam-

139

ily participation in a highly emotional human experience, with the result that home deliveries, with their attendant hazards for mother and infant, are growing in popularity.

The alternative birth center at Mount Zion Hospital and Medical Center seeks to respond to the need to broaden the spectrum of services for maternal and infant care, modifying traditional practices as needed to provide a more natural, human experience within an atmosphere that is satisfying to young couples and consistent with safe and preventive perinatal care.

This will be accomplished by:

1. Provision of a room in which the mother may labor and deliver her infant, supported and assisted by the father and other support people, in a nontraditional environment that can be personalized to their satisfaction, without obtrusive instrumentation and regimentation. Under specific guidelines, siblings may also be present for the birth.
2. The safety of mother and infant will be ensured by the presence of an obstetrical nurse throughout labor and delivery and by the availability of obstetrical and pediatric house staff at all times, with attending staff backup.
3. Immediate rooming-in and early discharge will be additional important features of the center's services, including careful examination of mother and infant and follow-up by home visits after discharge.

The policies and procedures that follow have been developed to provide uniform standards necessary to achieve these goals.

CRITERIA FOR ADMISSION

1. All patients must have prenatal supervision by a licensed physician, either a private attending obstetrician, clinic physician, or nurse-midwife under a physician's supervision.
2. No findings suggestive of increased risk of complications during labor, delivery, or immediate postpartum period should be present.
3. All patients must attend some type of prepared childbirth classes (Lamaze, Bradley, etc.).
4. All patients should participate in the orientation program for use of the alternative birth center provided by the Mount Zion staff.
5. All patients must understand that if their labor status changes to one of high risk, transfer to the regular labor and delivery area will be necessary.
6. All mothers who wish to use the center are expected to be accompanied by a support person.
7. All patients must sign an informed consent form accepting the risks involved in delivering in the alternative birth center prior to admission to the center.
8. A specific plan for family participation, if desired, must be agreed upon in advance.
9. The infant's pediatrician must be agreeable to the criteria for care of the newborn.

HIGH-RISK FACTORS EXCLUDING ADMISSION TO THE ALTERNATIVE BIRTH CENTER

A. Social factors
   1. Less than three prenatal visits
   2. Maternal age*
      a. Primipara more than 35 years old
      b. Multipara more than 40 years old

---

*Relative contraindication—may use center after period of fetal monitoring in the active phase of labor.

uid

rs

continuous fetal heart rate monitoring
complication that attending physician or nurse
osis or treatment than can be done in the alter-

N

together.

our

st if mother is Rh negative or blood type O

onnel, depending on time of day, ward schedule,
le

birth weight over 5 or under 9.5 pounds

97.7° to 99.5° F)

done by pediatric house officer or private pedia-

ix 45% or more
evidence of incompatibility
al observation
two formula or breastfeedings

4. Deeply stained meconium in amniotic fl
5. Abnormal fetal heart rate or pattern
6. Prolonged true labor, more than 24 hou
7. Arrest of labor in active phase
8. Second stage labor
   a. More than 2 hours for primigravida
   b. More than 1 hour for multiparas
9. Significant vaginal bleeding
10. Development of any factor that require
11. Any labor pattern or maternal or fetal
    feels requires more sophisticated diagn
    native birth center

CRITERIA FOR IMMEDIATE ROOMING-I

Mother and infant will remain in the cente
A. Initial evaluation of infant
   1. Five-minute Apgar 7 or over
   2. Weight over 5 or under 9.5 pounds
   3. Vital signs normal
      a. Heart rate 110 to 170
      b. Respirations 35 to 70
   4. Color normal
   5. Airway open, including nares
   6. Vitamin K given
   7. Erythromycin opthalmic ointment
   8. Papers completed
B. Observation period (4 to 6 hours)
   1. Frequent observations during first h
   2. Vital signs qh × 4, then q4h
   3. Hematocrit, Dextrostix at 4 hours
   4. Blood type, Coombs test, and Rh te
   5. Nurse present for first feeding
   6. Visitors at discretion of hospital pers
      space available, and number of peop

CRITERIA FOR EARLY DISCHARGE

A. Infant (between 10 A.M. and 10 P.M.)
   1. Not less than 6 hours post-partum
   2. Vital signs stable
      a. Temperature 36.5° to 37.5° C (
      b. Heart rate 110 to 160
      c. Respirations 30 to 60
   3. Physical examination normal; to b
      trician
   4. Hematocrit 45% to 65%; Dextrost
   5. Blood type, Coombs test show no
   6. No complication requiring additio
   7. At least one water feeding and/or

8. Mother must demonstrate ability to handle and care for infant
9. Birth certificate complete
10. Home care record understood; parents maintain notes of
    a. First voiding if not in hospital; notify if not by 24 hours
    b. First meconium stool; if not by 36 hours, notify
    c. Feedings
    d. Any changes in infant
11. Home visit to be made by nurse in first 24 hours and on day 3; on day 3 visit, nurse will draw blood to determine presence of PKU and bilirubin if indicated, or mother may take infant to pediatric clinic or private pediatrician

B. Mother
1. No medical complications requiring close supervision (e.g., cardiovascular problems, diabetes)
2. No antepartum or intrapartum obstetric complications requiring close postpartum observation (e.g., toxemia, hemorrhage, signs of infection)
   a. Length of labor
      (1) Less than 30 hours, primigravida
      (2) Less than 24 hours, multigravida
   b. Ruptured membranes, less than 24 hours
   c. Perineum: episiotomy or less than third-degree laceration with no additional vaginal or cervical lacerations, hematoma formation, or unusually severe bruising
   d. Blood loss less than 500 ml
   e. Delivery spontaneous or low forceps
   f. Analgesia/anesthesia: mother with spinal, caudal, epidural, or general anesthesia may not be discharged in less than 24 hours
3. Postpartum course
   a. Vital signs
      (1) Temperature less than 38° C (100.4° F)
      (2) Pulse less than 100
      (3) Blood pressure > 90/60, < 140/90, and consistent with prenatal course
   b. Fundus firm with no excessive bleeding
   c. Hematocrit more than 32% or hemoglobin more than 10.5 g/100 ml
   d. Able to ambulate easily and care for self and baby
   e. Able to void adequately
   f. RhoGAM eligibility determined, and plan for administration developed
   g. Plan for assistance at home for at least 2 days

NURSING PROCEDURES FOR THE ALTERNATIVE BIRTH CENTER
Admission procedures

A. Objectives
1. Provide supportive care to minimize stress of transition to the center during labor
2. Ensure optimal comfort of mother and support persons
3. Screen sibling, support persons, and any others for infectious conditions
B. General
1. Greet and assist family in making themselves comfortable
2. Obtain prenatal record, check for informed consent, review family preference sheet
3. Evaluate baseline labor status and psychologic factors; provide information and support as needed

    4. Notify physician, if not present, of patient's arrival; obtain orders and prepare patient for evaluation, including reviewing orders with the laboring mother
    5. Notify admitting office
    6. Screen siblings and exclude if temperature is over 37.2° C (99° F), or if cough, rhinitis, sore throat, skin lesions, or diarrhea is evident
    7. Screen others for obvious signs of infection
C. Procedures
    1. Follow physicians' orders and chart time and procedures on nurses' notes, including completion of admission note with age, gravidity, parity, estimated date of confinement (EDC), status of labor, show, baseline information, breast or bottle feeding
    2. Transpose admission information to graphic record, delivery record, newborn record, admission log, baby bands, birth certificate
    3. Ask patient to sign newborn identification; witness and complete
    4. Check family summary/preference sheet
    5. Draw routine blood work—CBC, VDRL, "hold clot"

Newborn early discharge

A. Maintain body temperature with body heat and/or warm blankets and heat lamps
B. Vitamin K_1 oxide (Aquamephyton), 1 mg intramuscularly
C. Vital signs qh × 4, then q4h
D. Blood type and Coombs test on cord blood if mother is type O or Rh negative.
E. VDRL on cord blood if mother's VDRL is reactive
F. Feeding
    1. Formula routine: 5% glucose in water q4h × 3, then formula
    2. Breast routine: to breast as soon as possible
G. Dextrostix at 4 hours
H. Hematocrit (heel stick) at 4 hours
I. Bacitracin to cord
J. Erythromycin ophthalmic ointment to both eyes
K. Determine presence of PKU prior to discharge or arrange to draw on third day home visit

Discharge orders—home care

A. Discharge infant and mother after all blood work and physical examinations have been completed
B. Evaluation by RN at home on days 1 and 3
C. Vital signs at visit
D. Check for PKU on third day by RN at home
E. Evaluate for signs of jaundice, and draw bilirubin if jaundiced
F. Record time of first urination; report to pediatrician if not in 24 hours
G. Record time of first meconium stool; report to pediatrician if not within 48 hours
H. Call pediatrician if any abnormalities, or after second visit if all is well

Home visits

A. General
    1. Discharge criteria completed for both mother and baby by nurse or patient coordinator before family leaves the hospital

    2. Birth certificate completed either by the hospital or at home, facilitated by the nurse

B. Home visit checks—baby
    1. Baby assessments, days 1 and 3
        a. Temperature
            (1) Axillary, normal range: 36.5° to 37.5° C (97.7° to 99.5° F)
            (2) Check extremities for touch, temperature, color
        b. Heart
            (1) Take apical pulse, normal range 110 to 160
            (2) Listen for heart sounds; normally only two heart sounds are heard
        c. Respirations
            (1) Watch chest for 1 full minute for respiratory rate
            (2) Check for signs of respiratory distress
            (3) Normal range 30 to 60
            (4) Listen for congested lungs; listen through back; ordinarily only hear breathing sounds
        d. Blood
            (1) Check for jaundice, draw blood to determine presence of bilirubin if needed
            (2) Indicate at each visit
        e. Cord
            (1) Normal is dry, falls off in 7 to 10 days
            (2) Indicate and check for moistness, odor, redness, granuloma, bleeding
        f. Circumcision: some staining unusual
        g. Breastfeeding
            (1) Evaluate as to number of feedings per 24-hour period, length of nursing on each breast, quality of suck
            (2) Check mother's milk flow, condition of nipples and breasts
            (3) Determine number of supplementary feedings, what, how many ounces, when offered
        h. Bottlefeeding: determine number of feedings, what, how many ounces, when offered
        i. Weight
            (1) Day of discharge for comparative purposes
            (2) Obtain weight on day 3 and prn
        j. Alertness, responsiveness should also be noted
        k. A complete physical assessment should be given to the baby by the nurse some time during the first few days; other aspects of physical assessment will vary according to findings on individual babies
    2. PKU: on day 3 draw blood to determine presence
    3. Bath demonstration, especially for primipara, in hospital or on day 3
    4. Parent education and support
        a. Be sure to discuss signs of illness with parents and how to obtain help, i.e., private pediatrician, emergency room, pediatric clinic; signs include changes in behavior, feeding patterns, elevated temperature, diarrhea, jaundice, respiratory distress
        b. If signs of distress are present, call pediatrician or pediatric house officer to report findings
        c. Let the family know you are available for advice at any time, especially through the first 2 weeks; you know this family and are in the best position to advise them appropriately

    d. Many of the nurse's interventions are directed toward parentcraft and helping the family make the transition into parenthood

C. Home visit checks—mother
1. Mother's examinations, days 1 and 3
    a. Temperature, pulse, respiration
      (1) If temperature is above 38° C (100.4° F) consult physician
      (2) Elevations of pulse or respiratory rate may be related to other changes
      (3) Normally, in the early postpartum period, the pulse rate may be increased to 90 to 100 per minute
      (4) Irregular cardiac rhythms may be initially noted with careful taking of radial pulse
    b. Blood pressure: normal between 90/60 and 140/90
    c. Breasts
      (1) Check for softness or firmness
      (2) Check for colostrum to milk
      (3) Check for tenderness, cracked or fissured nipples, lumps or hardened areas
      (4) Advise for tenderness, breast care
    d. Costovertebral angles
      (1) Normally no tenderness
      (2) If tender, check for signs of urinary difficulties
    e. Calves: normally no tenderness
    f. Perineum
      (1) Check episiotomy for separation, swelling, pain, infection; advise accordingly
      (2) Check lochia; normal findings:
        (a) Color: rubra by 1 to 2 days; brownish red by 2 to 4 days; serosanguineous by 2 to 7 days; alba after 7 to 10 days
        (b) Amount: if saturates pad in 2 hours (spots other side of pad after 12 hours post partum), then bleeding is too heavy
        (c) Some clots are normal, may be associated with cramping
        (d) Some breakthrough bright-red bleeding is normal through a few weeks after delivery if associated with increased activity or breastfeeding
        (e) Odor: resembles menses; foul odor may indicate infection
        (f) Advise as indicated by signs or symptoms; consult physician if abnormal
    g. Fundus
      (1) At umbilicus day of delivery; progresses to four to five fingerbreadths below umbilicus and well into the pelvis by 7 days
      (2) If above umbilicus or to the side, bladder may be full
      (3) Size of grapefruit initially, then progressively smaller
    h. Bowel movements: should have a bowel movement by day 3 post partum
    i. Voiding: check to see that mother is voiding without retention
    j. Do other aspects of a physical examination as indicated by concerns, signs, or symptoms
2. Call patient's physician or obstetric resident to report findings
3. Mother's postpartum appointment: remind her to make her appointment with her obstetrician or clinic
4. Review signs of illness with mother and how to obtain assistance
5. Review birth control methods
6. Remind mother you are available for advice, especially during first 3 days

MOUNT ZION HOSPITAL AND MEDICAL CENTER
San Francisco, California

Baby: _____

Hospital no.: _____

ALTERNATIVE BIRTH CENTER CHECKLIST

Mother: _____

HOME VISIT—DAY

Date: _____

General appearance

Color: Pink ☐   Dusky ☐   Cyanotic ☐   Jaundice ☐

Tone: Appropriate ☐   Poor ☐   Exaggerated ☐

Skin: Hydration _____   Marks _____

Head

Circumference _____   Molding _____   Fontanels _____

Abnormalities _____

Eyes: Discharge ☐   Nose: Patent ☐

Chest

Heart: Rate _____   Regular ☐   Irregular ☐

Respiration: Rate _____   Periodic ☐   Retractions ☐   Flaring ☐

Breath sounds _____

Abdomen

Umbilicus: Dry ☐   Red ☐   Draining ☐   Off ☐   On ☐

Contour _____   Masses _____

Genitals

Sex _____   Testes _____   Discharge _____

Circumcision: Healing ☐   Draining ☐

Extremities

ROM _____   Symmetric _____   Hip check _____   Deformities _____

Neurologic

Cry: Strong ☐   Weak ☐

Reflexes: Moro ☐   Blink ☐   Rooting ☐   Suck ☐

Feeding

Breast ☐   Bottle ☐   Duration _____   Quality _____   Satisfaction _____

Supplements _____

Bladder/bowel

Time first stool _____   Frequency _____   Color _____   Consistency _____

Voiding _____   PKU _____   Bilirubin _____

Assessment and recommendation:

_____

Signed

CERTIFIED NURSE-MIDWIVES

I. Definition

The nurse-midwife is a registered nurse who, by virtue of added knowledge and skill gained through an organized program of study and clinical experience recognized by the American College of Nurse-Midwives, has extended the limits (legal limits in jurisdictions where they pertain) of her practice into the area of management of care of mothers and babies throughout the maternity cycle, so long as progress meets criteria accepted as normal. Her education prepares the nurse-midwife to recognize deviations from normal at a time when medical care can be instituted to safeguard the well-being of the mother and her baby.

II. Minimum qualifications

A. Current licensure as a registered nurse in California.

B. Completion of a nurse-midwifery program approved by the American College of Nurse-Midwives.

C. Certification by examination by the American College of Nurse-Midwives.

D. Current license as a nurse-midwife in California.

E. Agreement for physician backup by a board-certified or board-eligible obstetrician in good standing on the staff of Mount Zion Hospital.

III. Criteria for nurse-midwifery management

The nurse-midwife may assume responsibility for the management of the obstetric care of patients who meet the following general criteria:

A. Medical, surgical, and past obstetric history reveals no condition that would adversely affect or be adversely affected by pregnancy.

B. No indication of current pathology present in mother, fetus, or newborn.

C. No obstetric findings present that are likely to require operative delivery.

IV. General policies

A. The nurse-midwife functions within the department of obstetrics gynecology, and the physician under whose direction the nurse-midwife is functioning must be indicated on the admission plate for the patient.

B. In her practice, the nurse-midwife will follow the guidelines established by the American College of Nurse-Midwives through the *Statements of Functions, Standards, and Qualifications for the Practice of Nurse-Midwives*.

C. Approved nurse-midwifery orders shall be available in all areas (labor and delivery, alternative birth center, and post partum); any order by a nurse-midwife, if written according to and within the listings of the approved nurse-midwifery orders, will receive the same attention by the nursing staff as if written by a physician; however, any order that is not within this listing must be countersigned by a physician before the nurse is permitted to carry out the order; all drug orders will be reviewed and countersigned by the consulting physician.

D. The criteria for normal, established by the Department of Obstetrics and Gynecology and the nursing service, shall be available in all areas.

E. Upon identification of deviations from normal progress, the nurse-midwife will consult with the obstetrician; findings and dispositions resulting from such consultation are to be charted by the nurse-midwife in the patient's record, or the physician will write a note of his own.

F. Collaborative care and/or transfer to medical management: upon diagnosis of obstetric or medical complications exceeding the limitations of nurse-midwifery practice,

MOUNT ZION HOSPITAL AND MEDICAL CENTER
San Francisco, California

Hospital no.: _____
Name of mother: _____

ALTERNATIVE BIRTH CENTER HOME VISIT CHECKLIST

POSTPARTUM DAY 1 Date: _____

Temperature, pulse, respiration
Blood pressure
Breast: Soft Filling Engorged Colostrum Milk
Nipples: OK Sore Cracked Inverted Flat
Fundus: Firm Boggy Soft Midline Umbilicus
Episiotomy/laceration: OK Separated Red Swollen
  Drain Gas copious Pain BM Heat Sitz
Lochia: Rubra Brown-red Serosang Alba Light
  Medium Heavy Clots Infected

Birth control plans

Medication:
Voiding: QS Burning pain
BM: Yes No Consistency Pain Bleed Med.
Extremities: Not tender Tender
Discussion: Infant care Exercise Diet

POSTPARTUM DAY 3 Date: _____

Temperature, pulse, respiration
Blood pressure
Breast: Soft Filling Engorged Colostrum Milk
Nipples: OK Sore Cracked Inverted Flat
Fundus: Firm Boggy Soft Midline Umbilicus
Episiotomy/laceration: OK Separated Red Swollen
  Drain Gas copious Pain BM Heat Sitz
Lochia: Rubra Brown-red Serosang Alba Light
  Medium Heavy Clots Infected

-0- Pill IUD Condom Foam Rhythm Diaphragm

Medication:
Voiding: QS Burning pain
BM: Yes No Consistency Pain Bleed Med.
Extremities: Not tender Tender
Discussion: Infant care Exercise Diet

Remarks and recommendations:

Abnormals and teaching should be explained in remarks _____

Signed _____

the patient will be transferred to medical management, but the nurse-midwife may continue to care for the patient as a skilled professional nurse under the direction of the physician.

V. Approved procedures

  A. Intrapartum. The nurse-midwife will:

   1. Evaluate the patient's labor status, authorize admission, and write appropriate admitting orders.

   2. Initiate and manage nonstress test and oxytocin challenge tests following physician consultation or direction.

   3. Initiate and manage oxytocin induction or augmentation following physician consultation or direction.

   4. Provide support and nursing management of complicated patients under physician management; under certain circumstances, such patients' infants may be delivered by the nurse-midwife following mutual agreement between the nurse-midwife and the physician.

   5. Manage the labor and delivery of patients who meet criteria accepted as normal.

THE FAMILY BIRTH CENTER, LOS GATOS (CALIFORNIA) COMMUNITY HOSPITAL

Anthony J. Damore, M.D.

Perhaps the first question asked about family birth centers is, "Why even consider a new method of delivery in a small community hospital where maternity care has traditionally been accepted as being provided in a safe and adequate manner?" When considering the numerous obstacles involved in setting up such a program, the question "why" becomes even more intriguing. These obstacles can be divided into nonmedical and medical categories.

Nonmedical barriers

In our case the most difficult nonmedical barrier was the hospital administration. Regardless of the most convincing arguments for change in the hospital structure, the final decision was, as is usual, influenced by the economic picture. Although family birth centers (FBCs) may not be designed to make money for the hospital, they *are* designed to be more efficient and thus not lose money. In addition, birth centers can lower the cost of hospital maternity care for the family. Traditionally, a childbearing family uses a labor room, a delivery room, and a postpartum room, with personal care required in each of these separate areas. This routine requires a lot of increasingly expensive materials and personnel. Consider now the birth center: a single room for labor, delivery, and recovery, with a single nurse in continuous attendance. The couple and their support persons are encouraged to be self-sufficient in attending to their nonmedical needs. In terms of reducing the amount of materials and number of staff required, the birth center does make good economic sense.

Other concerns of the hospital administration were accreditation and public opinion. The California State Health Department licensing division had strong feelings about what was placed on the walls and floors of the room. Also, traffic patterns, general procedures, rules, regulations, safety measures, and other details needed approval. I found the health department licensing division most cooperative and helpful as these issues were systematically resolved.

In dealing with public opinion, cautious innovation while anticipating problems was the key to success. The hospital auxiliary was most helpful in publicizing the birth center, as well as in decorating it. In fact, one of the first things we did was have special meetings with the auxiliary to familiarize them with the birth center and answer their numerous questions.

Medical barriers

After the nonmedical barriers were removed, we began to deal with the medical barriers, which meant many staff meetings. Everyone involved with the birth center had a part in its formation, including childbirth educators in the area, all the obstetric and pediatric RNs and LVNs/LPNs, the hospital nursing office, the infection control committee, and the obstetricians and pediatricians. Local nurse-midwives and lay midwives were invited to our first few meetings to discuss home births in our community. This interaction was very informative for hospital staff and those working in the community. After numerous meetings, we began to identify the feelings, ideas, and facts that would ultimately form our official rules and regulations governing the birth center.

The physicians were the most resistant to change because they were not convinced of the need for such a center. Many felt uncomfortable in a new setting without electronic fetal monitors and other medical devices. There are still several physicians on the staff who use the birth center reluctantly, and then only because of consumer pressure to do so.

After both nonmedical and medical barriers to our birth center were dealt with, we turned our attention to the minute details of development.

The room

Selecting an appropriate room for the birth center was not difficult. We wanted something private and out-of-the-way yet close enough to traditional areas for needed emergency intervention. We converted a two-bed postpartum room at the end of a hall, which provides an ideal closed-traffic pattern. The room is spacious enough to allow the couple and their support persons to move about in a comfortable, relaxed manner, yet maintains a sense of privacy with the intimacy of a family gathering. Once decided on, the room was stripped of all traditional hospital wall and ceiling fixtures, leaving only the oxygen line. Refurnishing and redecorating

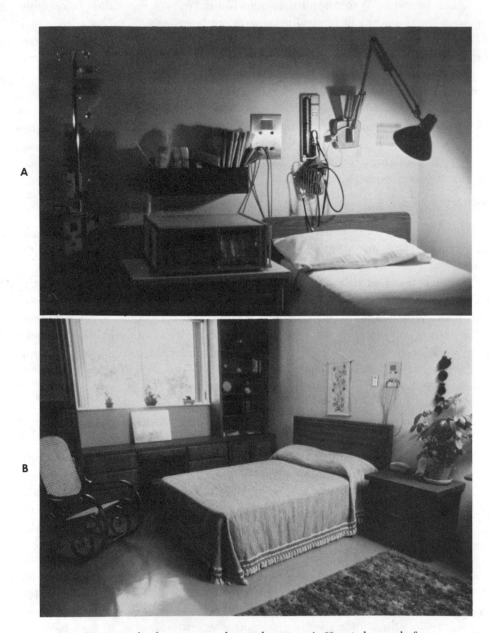

Fig. 7-1. An alternative birth center in a hospital setting. **A,** Hospital room before conversion. **B,** After conversion.

were done in a practical, thoughtful, and medically acceptable manner. Input from the nurses, physicians, and infection control committee was considered.

The new wall covering was the first and probably the most important consideration. We decided on a floor-to-ceiling mural (Fig. 7-2) covering two adjoining walls opposite the head of the bed. It is a summer forest scene that seems to encircle the room with colors which are cool and relaxing. Bright spots of sun filtering through the trees offer numerous points of fixation for concentration during labor. On the wall adjacent to the headboard is the oxygen outlet, along with wall hangings, pictures, plants, and other decorations. There is a floor-to-ceiling wall unit on either side of the window, with a large desk area under the window, useful to nurses, physicians, and patients. These units were nicely finished and house all the needed medical and housekeeping supplies. Decorative blinds are used on the window because of the ease of cleaning and adjustment for light control.

The bed selected was a normal double bed with a wooden headboard and no side rails or footboard, thus permitting ease of movement onto and off the bed. A protective plastic case is used for the mattress and box spring, and the frame is elevated to facilitate manipulation during delivery and any postpartum repairs. A decorative spread, which is removed once active labor begins, adds to the homey atmosphere. All lighting is provided by floor lamps. The delivery is accomplished using a directional beam, which permits localization of the lighting without any unnecessary brightness and glare.

The birth center has an independent thermometer, which is adjusted at delivery to about 26.7° C (80° F). This permits the couple to freely touch, hold, and communicate with their newborn without fear of the baby's temperature dropping. We did several studies on skin and rectal temperatures of infants delivered in the traditional setting as compared with those in the birth center. There were strong variations of temperature with the traditional methods but few, if any, variations in the birth center babies.

In the corner of the room is a sofa that has multiple uses. Visiting support persons, sleeping fathers, and doting new grandparents have all found the sofa comfortable and practical. A bentwood rocking chair, originally placed in the room as an amenity, has proved to be a favorite of nursing mothers and pampering fathers. Rugs, plants, books, radio, and record player all add that special homelike touch.

As the room was undergoing transformation, so too were our feelings and ideas about childbirth. While compiling an outline of rules and regulations to govern the usage of the FBC, we became increasingly more involved; the key words seemed to always be involvement and commitment.

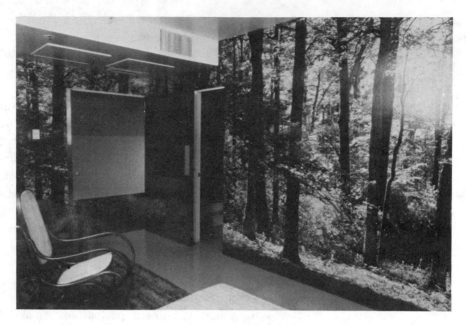

Fig. 7-2. Floor-to-ceiling mural.

Staff

Those who became involved in the FBC had to make a commitment. The physicians were pledged to provide a safe medical environment for mother and baby within the center. Sometimes this requires more effort and cooperation than with traditional methods because the focal point here is the mother in labor, not the convenience of the physician. Many times it is physically harder to deliver babies and do episiotomy repairs when the woman is in a bed. It may take longer to let a patient completely expel the baby spontaneously than to assist birth with outlet forceps. It can be quite uncomfortable working in a 26.6° C (80° F) room. The nurses are kept busy helping the women move around and change position, directing the support persons, completing all the extra paperwork, attending to nursing duties, but above all being there with the couple all the time, trying to be cheerful, helpful, and supportive. There is extra effort involved compared with the traditional routine blood pressure and fetal heart tone (FHT) checks and periodic cervical examinations. Often after the delivery, the nurse looks like she, too, went through labor.

Is all this extra effort worthwhile? Indeed it is because even the most stouthearted antagonist experiences something new and exciting during a FBC delivery.

There is a different type of electricity in the air, and the childbearing woman is the catalyst. The emotional intensity sometimes reaches such a peak during delivery that it seems to envelope everyone. This intimate time is not, and should not be, interrupted by moving the labor bed to a delivery room, moving to a delivery table, getting into stirrups, or listening to directions from physicians and nurses. It is a time when all involved concentrate on the task at hand and lend support and encouragement to the mother.

Preparation

The couple's involvement begins early in pregnancy with childbirth education classes, a basic requirement for usage of the family birth center. Included in the classes are discussions on nutrition, basic anatomy and physiology, and breathing exercises to help the couple better understand and cope with pregnancy, labor, and delivery. During this time the couples are encouraged to take one of the routinely scheduled tours through the hospital birth center. By visiting the center couples seem better able to relate plans for their delivery, to the actual experience. After completing these classes the couple must attend a FBC orientation class. This is a one-evening class when movies and slides of family birth center births are shown. There are discussions and talks on related subjects, such as anesthesia, episiotomy, circumcision, and breastfeeding. The couples are given forms to be completed by their obstetrician and pediatrician, which formalize their agreement to follow the center's rules and regulations. The couple is asked to complete a preference list, which itemizes their preferences and plans for usage of the family birth center. As much as possible, these requests are complied with at the time of labor and birth.

Labor

When labor starts the woman comes to the hospital, where she is evaluated by a nurse to be sure that she is in labor and not at risk. If the woman was identified as high risk prenatally, she should already have been screened out of the birth center, since only uncomplicated cases can deliver there. If no problems have developed since the last prenatal visit and everything is uncomplicated, the woman in labor is then admitted to the family birth center. Once in the center she is given freedom and usage of the room as predetermined by her preference sheet. If she has elected to have siblings present, there must be a separate support person to continuously care for them, but they are permitted ingress and egress at the couple's discretion. Sibling presence is discussed at length during the classes, and appropriate screening and education is done at that time.

Some prefer to stand and walk when in active labor, whereas others prefer different positions in bed. When active labor begins, the women usually get into bed, often reclining in the arms of their husbands, who sit behind them, giving help and support. We have found that this seems to be the best position for the father, since it allows privacy for communication and closeness for touching and sharing.

Delivery

The floor lights are dimmed, if desired, and the delivery is usually accomplished in the sitting partial lithotomy position, although delivery can be and has been accomplished in the lateral Sims position, kneeling on all fours, or even the knee-chest position. Once the baby begins to emerge, the couple is encouraged to touch the child and help in the emergence. As soon as completely born, the infant is placed on the mother's bare abdomen with the cord intact. A warm blanket is then placed over the infant, and breast feeding is encouraged. While the couple is getting acquainted with their new infant, the perineal area is inspected, and any needed suturing accomplished. By this time the cord usually has stopped pulsating, and the father is encouraged to assist in actually cutting the cord. Also, by this time the placenta has usually separated and been delivered. Everything is cleaned up, and other people in the room are encouraged to get more involved if they have not so far, although during the active stages of labor everyone usually is quite involved, offering encouragement to the mother while she breathes and pushes. Once the baby is born, everyone joins in with cheers and congratulations. That is the way a birthday should be! The baby stays with the family in the room until discharge.

Early discharge

Early discharge is a family birth center option, and if medically safe the family is free to leave when they feel ready. Most early discharges occur about 6 to 12 hours post partum, since by that time the woman has voided, ambulated, and eaten something, and the uterus is firm and the lochia acceptable. Everyone who elects discharge prior to 24 hours automatically has a home visit by one of our maternity nurses within the next 24 hours. At the home visit checks on mother and baby are performed as needed. Lab tests are done, a verbal report is forwarded to the physician, and a written report made part of the chart. If desired or needed, a second home visit can also be made at 72 hours. The quality and quantity of the time spent depend specifically on the individual needs of the patient.

Only uncomplicated pregnancies are admitted to the family birth center, and if complications develop during the labor or delivery, the woman must be transferred to the traditional areas for treatment. IV infusions, electronic fetal monitors, prepartum oxytocics, conduction anesthesia (except paracervical and/or pudendal blocks), forceps, and excessive analgesics are not permitted in the family birth center. If the problem requiring transfer is resolved, the woman can be readmitted. Families are instructed and encouraged to use the center either alone or in any combination with the delivery room and postpartum rooms. For example, some women with complicated pregnancies can labor with monitors, etc., in the labor room, deliver in the delivery room, but then recover in the family birth center.

Summary

After our first year we were concerned about whether we had achieved our family birth center goals. We have a guest book into which FBC couples make entries at the time of delivery. These responses have been overwhelmingly positive but certainly could be colored by enthusiasm from the recent delivery. Months later, however, a truer picture of the value of the family birth center might emerge. To get appropriate feedback we decided to have a 1-year FBC party to which we invited all the FBC families and their friends.

Our expectations were exceeded. We were first of all impressed with the show of people, especially those who had to make special arrangements to come. In general their comments reflected the feeling that the delivery provided a special, lasting, positive influence on the family because of the family birth center. We were suspicious that any first delivery might be viewed this way, so we especially sought out comments from multiparous patients. It did not seem to matter. Parents of diverse backgrounds, number of children, ages, number of support persons— they all had similar comments. Yes! The family birth center was successful. We had provided a safe, humanistic, fulfilling, and memorable birth experience.

The family birth center has been operating since 1978, and the deliveries have been slowly increasing, although interestingly enough our total number of deliveries has not significantly changed. It seems that we are not attracting that many new patients, but the women who are using the hospital are switching from traditional methods to the family birth center. It is difficult to assess the future of the center, but it seems reasonable in this era of diminishing birthrates not to measure the success or failure of a birth center merely on number of deliveries. The true value and success of the family birth center is in the redefinition of childbirth, its setting, and the attitudes involved. Childbirth should be thought of as a nondisease process completed under nonhospital conditions with participation by interested, sensitive people. Childbirth, with its work and responsibilities, has been returned to the couples. Decision making is more of a joint venture, with the medical team observing from the sidelines, supporting and giving assistance when needed or requested, making medical decisions when indicated. This is not a step down for the medical and nursing professions; it is a maturing of their roles as they realize that childbirth is an event which should be participated in to the fullest by those involved, yet directed and guided by medical people for a safe, rewarding experience. There can be no question that parturition has entered a new era for those who have come into contact with the family birth center and its philosophy.

The following statistics show the number of women using the family birth center at the end of one year.

A. Began labor in FBC—196
B. Deliveries—135
   1. Nullipara—72
   2. Multipara—63
C. Dropouts for medical reasons—61 (31%, or ⅓)
   1. Cesarean section—30
   2. Labor bed delivery—4
   3. Delivery room delivery—27
      a. IV—6
      b. Toxemia—2
      c. Premature—3
      d. Fetal distress—4
      e. Bleeding—2
      f. "By choice"—4
      g. Delivery prior to class—3
      h. Developed fever—1
      i. Twins—1
      j. Caudal anesthesia—1

BIRTH ROOM, DOMINICAN HOSPITAL, SANTA CRUZ, CALIFORNIA
Joseph T. Anzalone, M.D.

"Alternative birth": in most obstetricians these two words will bring forth a response of either fear or anger. "Alternative to what?" I have heard. "Surely not our markedly improving maternal and perinatal mortality. Could any alternative to our traditional type of birth offer the same protections to mother and baby?"

The idea of a homelike atmosphere in which a woman could labor had crossed my mind on many occasions in the past, but it was not until I visited the Mount Zion Alternative Birth Center in San Francisco that the idea was brought into full perspective. There, a room in the maternity suite offers all the comforts of one's own bedroom with the safety of still being in a hospital.

I agree we have progressed since the dark ages when fathers were relegated to their own special waiting room, and often, with the right combination of drugs, even the mother was eliminated while the physician delivered the baby. Still, our traditional labor and delivery rooms are cluttered and uncomfortable. Pregnancy is a time of great dependence for most women, who are traditionally placed in an unfamiliar room filled with objects they do not readily identify with while in labor, intensifying their feelings.

Labor beds are frequently firmer and narrower than most other hospital beds, making turning or assuming a comfortable position difficult. The narrow beds often necessitate the use of side rails, which make many women feel caged.

It is hard to imagine anyone not accepting a warmer, more comfortable, home-like area to labor. If the pregnancy and labor are uncomplicated, why not allow families to give birth in this friendly, private space? The "why not" was never answered, but opposition to birth rooms from several obstetricians on our staff was considerable.

An alternative birth center opened at a nearby community hospital, and two effects quickly became apparent: women who probably would have given birth at home began once again to elect delivery in the hospital; and the competition caused our hospital obstetrics program to begin to decline.

Over the next year many proposals were made, and finally, with hospital administration mediation, a compromise was worked out using a birthing room concept and the Borning Beds. These rooms, just like alternative birthing rooms, offer the family a comfortable private space for childbirth from the time they enter the hospital until they go home. The Borning Bed has the ability to "break," so the

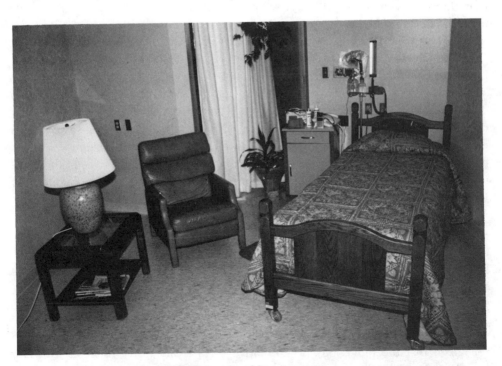

Fig. 7-3. Comfortable private space.

patient can quickly be put into stirrups. Generally, this option is not used unless an episiotomy is performed or laceration occurs. Even in the unbroken mode a simple push of a button will cause the upper half of the bed to raise approximately 10 inches and allow the easy management of an unsuspected shoulder dystocia. I feel the safety of this bed far outweighs any additional comfort that a double bed may afford.

It is interesting to me that, although we started out from a different direction, what we have ended up with is a room very similar to that developed by Dr. Philip Sumner in Manchester, Connecticut. It is hoped that by using this simple and humanistic approach more hospitals will be able to minimize intervention and maximize the joys of childbirth.

ALTERNATIVE BIRTH CENTER, SANTA CRUZ (CALIFORNIA) COMMUNITY HOSPITAL
Joseph D'Amico, M.D.

I read of alternatives to traditional birth in the lay press while completing my residency at a large metropolitan medical center where no one ever practiced obstetrics in any way but traditionally, with medicated births. It was obvious to me that there were definite problems with medicated births in terms of infant outcome. When I sought a place to live and practice obstetrics, I found in Santa Cruz not only an ideal living environment, but also a community ready for alternatives to traditional birth practices. When I moved there, many of the childbearing people in the community were looking for a more humanistic approach to birth, and approximately 10% of them were choosing home births. A unique situation also existed in that the community hospital had an almost nonfunctioning obstetrics department, and consequently the hospital administration was willing to accept an innovative approach to maternity care in an attempt to revive the floundering department. With the help of nurses, childbirth educators, and midwives in the community, we began an alternative birth center (ABC) at the Santa Cruz Community Hospital about 6 months after I began private obstetric practice there.

The birthing population using the ABC grew by patient referral. People happy with their birth experiences quickly told others. In addition, the public relations department of the hospital worked hard to inform the community of the new center. Within 2 months the number of births had increased at Community Hospital, along with the support nurses and midwives. Their energy was vital as the concept grew. Nurses are the birth center; it is their enthusiasm that makes it work.

People who chose the ABC wanted a compromise to home birth that would be safe and at the same time offer a wonderul, joyous experience. It is important to recognize that the philosophy of alternative birth is not just a room in which to give birth but actually extends to the entire experience. If patients become high

Text continued on p. 166.

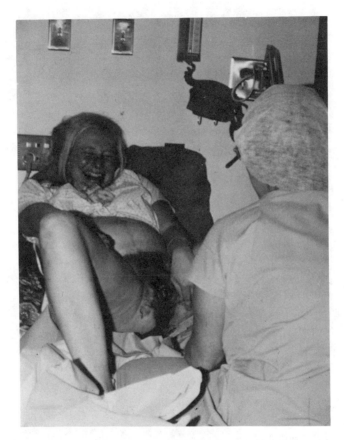

Fig. 7-4. Crowning.

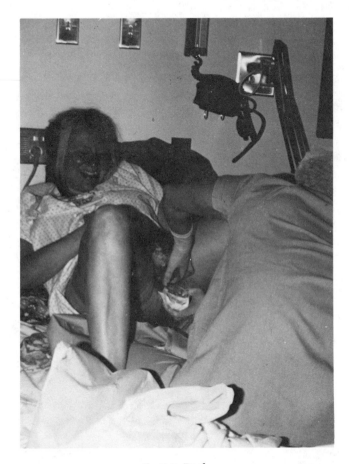

Fig. 7-5. Birth.

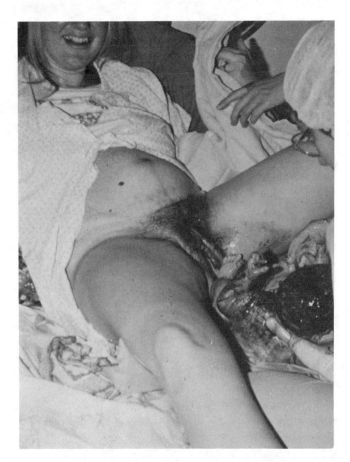

Fig. 7-6. A happy compromise to home birth.

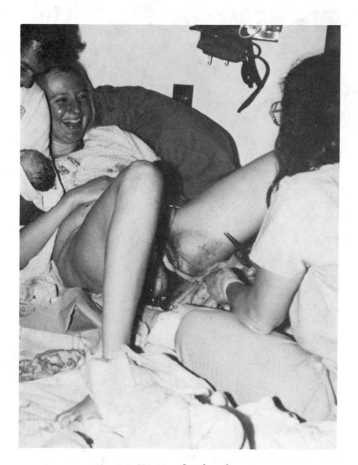

Fig. 7-7. Waiting for the placenta.

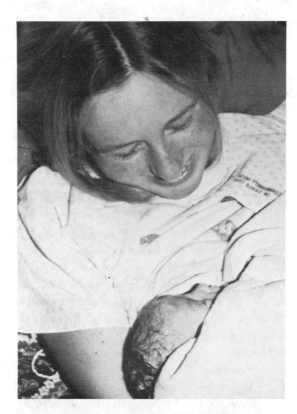

Fig. 7-8. Mother and baby.

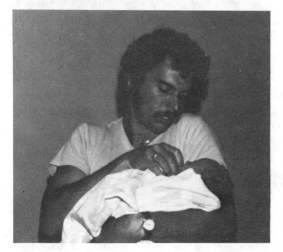

Fig. 7-9. Father and baby.

risk during labor and have to move from the ABC to a standard delivery room, that same philosophy of kindness and calmness follows them.

In the ABC setting technology is out of place. Bringing technology into the birth center creates a feeling that something is not quite right, so if there is any indication of problems, we try to move to a different setting. Thus the family is better able to accept necessary interventions, such as IV infusions or electronic fetal monitoring. Keeping the birth center for low-risk labors and births is vital to the concept of the center as a compromise between home and hospital births.

Couples using the ABC are able to have a great deal of control over their birth experiences. At this time, the decision to include siblings at the birth is usually made on an individual basis. There are insufficient data on which to base policies regarding the age at which siblings can attend births without long-term sequelae. It may be a long time before we have those data, so each family must decide for themselves about sibling participation in the birth.

There are some disadvantages for physicians in delivering babies in the low double bed in the birth room, such as the variety of often uncomfortable positions that one must maneuver into to deliver the baby and do perineal repair if necessary. It is always better to anticipate problems and move to a standard delivery room, if possible. Approximately 12% of the women admitted to the birth center are transferred during labor because of antepartum problems.

As use of the ABC increases it is becoming obvious that it is not a fad but a concept that is here to stay. People are returning for their second births in the ABC, and most who select my practice do so because of the birth center. The obstetrics census of 16 to 18 births a month when the ABC began has grown to 70 to 80 births a month. At times I am concerned about how to maintain the quality of care with this ever-increasing census. However, I feel that it is inevitable that the census will continue to grow. We began with one ABC room and now have four in use a great deal of the time. The alternative birth center is working and meeting the needs of this childbearing population.

THE CHILDBEARING CENTER, MATERNITY CENTER ASSOCIATION, NEW YORK

Ruth Watson Lubic, C.N.M.

We live in an age of active, informed consumerism. In increasing numbers childbearing families are seeking to expand their options in health care.

Maternity care

The term maternity care is used here to describe the physical monitoring and emotional support provided to families to ensure a safe and satisfying outcome of the childbearing cycle. The expectant mother is central to the process, and therefore the care is described as *maternity* care. Maternity care is health promoting and highly educative in nature. It also contributes to family cohesiveness, whether that family be consanguineous or fictive; ideally it is the mother who defines the "family" she wishes to be involved in her childbearing experience. Maternity care places high value on the feelings and attitudes of the family and on the humane behavior of attendants during childbirth. Maternity care fosters self-confidence in families in their role of bringing forth and rearing a child; it ensures the mother that she will have options and the opportunity to labor and give birth with dignity. Maternity care is also prototypically preventive mental health care in the sense that an individual's mental health begins with the mother's feelings and attitudes toward her pregnancy.

Obstetric care

It is inexact to use the term maternity care interchangeably with obstetric care, which is a provider-oriented description. Obstetric care is care provided by obstetricians; likewise nurse-midwifery care is care provided by nurse-midwives. If the childbearing experience deviates from normal, then obstetric care should be given priority over midwife or nonspecialist physician care; obstetric expertise is required for the management of complicated childbirths.

The use of an obstetric specialist functioning within his/her territory, the hospital, should not exclude a family-centered approach such as that of Dr. Sumner; however, apparently it often has if one can judge by the childbirth revolution raging both in the United States and abroad. In addition to the extensive upheaval in the United States* consumer dissatisfaction in Great Britain, France, Switzerland, Sweden, Canada, Australia, and New Zealand has been communicated to Maternity Center Association by professionals and families. Generally, depersonalization and routine intervention and surgery are the focuses of complaints.

Maternity care, then, can be defined as preventive, health-oriented management of the childbearing experience, with high value being accorded to cultural, emotional, and spiritual as well as physical needs of the family involved. Obstetric care is appropriately provided for those families whose childbearing is complicated; others less extensively prepared than obstetricians can provide care for healthy families.[12,13,15,19] Historically, physical needs have been given priority in the management of complicated childbearing. However, if public opinion can be taken as an indicator, it appears now that physical needs have often been given exclusive attention, and the management necessary for complicated births is being routinely applied to normal ones.

*See references 3, 4, 6, 9, 10, 12, 15, 18, 19, 21, and 24.

Alternative care

The word alternative is used here for forms of care other than the in-hospital management of parturition, which has been described by some families and in the literature as depersonalized, interventionist, authoritarian, and technologically oriented.* This section particularly explores the alternative known as a birth or childbearing center. Home birth is another alternative, as is the humanization of the inhospital setting.

In the United States in-hospital management of childbearing developed during this century and by the late 1960s had come to within 1% of being the universal method of management.[8] However, as recently as the 1930s almost half of American infants were still being born outside hospitals, for the most part in the parturient's home. The major movement into hospitals occurred during and following World War II; thus the incorporation of childbirth into a hospital setting has been comparatively recent and rapid. Maternity Center Association (MCA) joined the movement to encorage hospital births, as did other agencies and health professionals, on the theory that hospital care might provide the best insurance against mother and infant tragedies and loss. At the same time, however, MCA recognized the potential threat of routinization rather than individualization of services and worked hard to promulgate and maintain personalized care.

Alternative maternity care is a concept that includes more than merely the site in which care is given; much more important is the philosophy that the word alternative denotes, particularly the emphasis on health-, rather than illness-, oriented care. In such an orientation health workers other than specialized obstetric/gynecologic surgeons are the providers of choice. MCA has worked on the premise that these three aspects, health orientation, nonsurgical management, and out-of-hospital placement, are interdependent, but the complete potential of this interrelationship is not yet known. The likelihood of interdependence was important to the development of the Childbearing Center.

Maternity Center Association—agent for change

History. Maternity Center Association is a national voluntary health agency that provides an insitutional mechanism for dedicated women to influence and humanize birth practices in the United States. It was organized in 1917 to demonstrate a model of prenatal care.

From the beginning a vital part of the demonstration was parent education, although the content of classes has changed over the years. Initially mothers were motivated to come to the prenatal care centers because they were provided mate-

---

*See references 1, 2, 5, 7, 11, 25, and 26.

rials for layettes on which they sewed while advice on infant care, feeding, and health maintenance was given. Mothers were encouraged to attend to their own diets, and thus fetal well-being, through demonstrations of food preparation and the provision of nutritious meals. Fathers were always welcome, and special classes for fathers were organized in the 1930s. They became markedly more involved in the late 1940s with the advent of prepared childbirth. Dr. Grantly Dick-Read's book *Childbirth Without Fear*[23] was first published in Great Britain in 1942. When it came to MCA's attention, Dr. Dick-Read's humanistic concern and confidence that women could and would trust their bodies, if properly instructed, inspired MCA to invite him for a speaking tour of the United States.

MCA has prepared teaching materials for both professionals and the public. The film "Birth of a Baby," produced in 1937 with MCA's assistance, was a first in the field and was met with censorship by local police agencies. MCA's *Birth Atlas* continues to have worldwide distribution and use.

Nurse-midwifery education was introduced in the United States by MCA in 1931. However, the role of nurse-midwives was not acknowledged by organized obstetrics until 1970. A primary concern now in meeting the needs of childbearng families through nurse-midwifery care relates to the need for expanded and enriched educational programs.

MCA has been an effective agent for change in prenatal care, parent education, prepared childbirth, and nurse-midwifery education. Its secret is simple—focus on what families are saying they need and amalgamate that information with the best proven scientific health care practice.

The need for change. The first stirrings of the Childbearing Center (CbC) as a concept came in 1970 when MCA staff professionals detected a new determination in some childbearing couples to give birth out of the hospital. A causal hypothesis is that hospitals—or rather the professionals functioning within the hospitals—had grown increasingly insensitive to the desire of family members for each other's presence in times of crisis and celebration, particularly during and surrounding childbirth.

MCA responded to this childbirth revolution by attempting to meet the needs of both the families refusing to use the in-hospital system and the professionals from whom they felt alienated. Families need safety, satisfaction, and economy. Professionals have typically shown little concern for the family's satisfaction and have rationalized routinized behavior as being necessary for safe management.

The selection—a childbearing center

The decision was made to establish a free-standing birth center linked to the health care delivery system. It was felt that the birth center concept exhibited the greatest potential for providing safety, satisfaction, and economy. In MCA's opinion, economy would play a critical role because it affects both individual families and the system as a whole.

Description. The Childbearing Center was designed to provide a setting for maternity care that would be as homelike as possible and yet provide additional measures of safety. The starting point for design was home and not hospital, with emphasis placed on the fact that a childbearing center is *not* a minihospital. Every effort was made to eliminate or reduce the use of modalities that, although regarded as routine in hospital practice, carry risks. Oxytocin (Pitocin) induction or stimulation and forceps deliveries are examples; in our opinion, they should be used only in settings where remedies for their potential untoward effects are available.

To achieve this, the CbC was planned as an out-of-hospital unit in MCA's headquarters, formerly a private townhouse on East 92nd Street in New York. Space on two floors is used for the conduct of care. The entrance floor contains an office/reception room, waiting foyer, examination room, multipurpose room, private consultation room, and two rest rooms. Although most laboratory work is contracted out, there is a small laboratory containing a centrifuge and microscope. On the floor below is another examining room, a family room where early labor might be spent, and the intrapartum unit. Within the intrapartum unit are two birth rooms, utility rooms including an autoclave, a kitchen, two bathrooms, a shower/dressing room, and an alcove for emergency equipment. Families in early labor can also use the garden.

Care is provided by a staff medical team consisting of obstetricians, nurse-midwives, pediatricians, public health nurses, and ancillary personnel. (Nurse-midwife assistants were added to the team as the program got underway.) Families themselves are considered members of the decision-making team. Screening for physical health and childbirth education are two important facets of the program. A nearby hospital provides backup in emergencies, and visiting nurse public health nursing agencies contract to conduct follow-up home visits.

The CbC operates as a Diagnostic and Treatment Center under Article 28 of the New York State Public Health Law.

Process. The service begins when an interested family member inquires about it either in person or by telephone. At that time we screen out as ineligible for care at the center those mothers who (1) are 35 years old or older for first babies or 39 years old or older for a second through fourth delivery, (2) have had a cesarean section, (3) have a physical illness such as cardiac disease or diabetes, or (4) are more than 22 weeks pregnant. However, all families whether eligible or not are invited to attend an orientation, at which time the full operation of the center is discussed, pros and cons are considered, and questions answered. A tour of the facility is included.

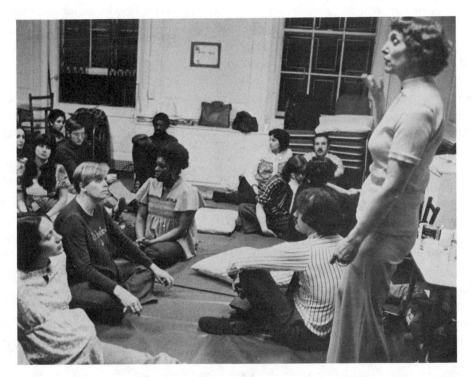

Fig. 7-10. Childbirth education. (Courtesy Maternity Center Association, Mariette Pathy Allen.)

Families are encouraged to think about the idea and discuss their plans with their gynecologist and other important persons before reaching a decision. When a family decides to have the physical screening, an appointment is made, and they are sent history forms, a general consent form, and other information about classes, fees, and so forth. On their first appointment a nurse-midwife reviews the forms with the family, and the consent form is signed. An obstetrician does the initial physical examination as well as a check-up examination at the thirty-sixth week. Other prenatal care is supervised by staff nurse-midwives.

Any deviation from normal calls for consultation with one of the obstetricians. Our philosophy is that families can adequately care for themselves when provided with principles and guidance. They must eventually care for their child; learning to take care of the fetus is the best preparation for this responsibility.

The family is accepted for care at the center with the understanding that re-screening will take place at every visit. Three early classes are scheduled: one on nutrition, one on touch and relaxation, and one on changes in pregnancy. Additional instruction in childbearing and infant care is required, either through self-care classes or more traditional classes, which are held separately.

The fee for comprehensive care is currently $1000 and enables the center to be self-supporting when an estimated 450 families enroll each year. The fee covers all charges, including professional care provided by the staff medical team. Circumcision is extra, as are any special tests such as an RH titration. MCA obstetricians serve as consultants when necessary and, if the family so desires, will act as backup in the event that transfer to a hospital becomes necessary. A decision about pediatric care must be made by the twenty-eighth week of pregnancy, even though our staff pediatrician sees the baby before the family leaves after childbirth.

When labor begins, families are encouraged to remain at home as long as they are comfortable in doing so. When they do come into the center, the mother is encouraged to be up and about with her family in the family room or garden. When the mother is admitted to one of the two labor/delivery rooms (Fig. 7-11), prepared family members, including children, may accompany her. Nurse-midwives assist the mother during delivery; obstetricians are not present. No routine procedures are used. The mothers labor in a position of comfort and deliver their infants in the labor bed.

Although available, analgesia is seldom used. Oral intake of fluids is encouraged, and families bring their own food for celebrating after the birth (Fig. 7-12). The healthy infant is never separated from the parents and may be cuddled and fed as they please. The pediatric examination is performed in the parents' presence.

Our experiences thus far have had a high degree of safety. We had had over 600 births at the center by early 1980. Currently about 10% of those who present themselves for intrapartum care require in-hospital management. (Failure to prog-

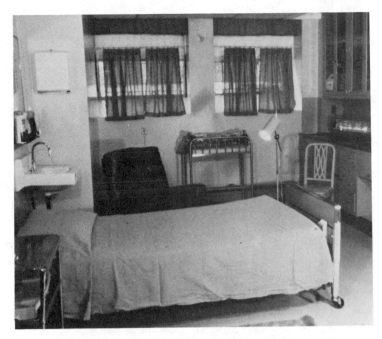

Fig. 7-11. Labor-delivery room. (Courtesy Maternity Center Association, Mariette Pathy Allen.)

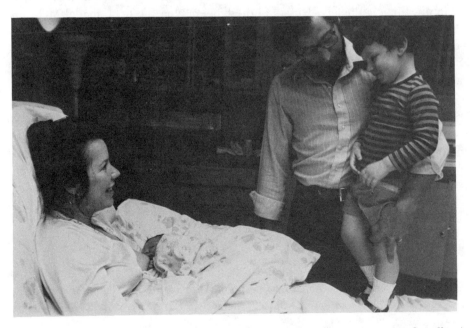

Fig. 7-12. After the birth. (Courtesy Maternity Center Association, Mariette Pathy Allen.)

Table 6. Event information—antepartum and intrapartum
(Oct. 1, 1975 to June 30, 1979)

Event		% (N = 1166)
First visit	1166	—
Ineligible first visit	101	8.7
Spontaneous abortion	42	3.6
Moved or withdrew	109	9.3
Referred or transferred	292	25.0
Delivered	455	39.0
Remaining in program	167	14.3

ress in labor, development of hypertension, and meconium staining are reasons for transfer to a hospital for care.) Approximately 65% of our parents are having their first child, and almost half are between the ages of 25 and 29 (Table 6).

To date, we have had none of the feared emergencies—abruptio placentae, cord prolapse, or postpartum hemorrhage. All mothers and infants transferred to the hospital in labor or post partum have done well.

The ripple becomes a wave

At the time of this writing there are some 40 to 50 birth centers known by us to be in operation nationally. Not all of these operate on the team model MCA promulgates, but all do seem to operate because of the same recurring circumstances—young families refusing to use hospital facilities.

Although the concept of a birth center may be innovative in our current hospital-oriented medical care system, it is certainly not a new idea and is an evident solution to the unattended home birth problem. The concept has been and will be used again and again as perceived needs arise. By the end of 1979 over 1300 professionals had actually visited the Childbearing Center; we have not tabulated the many telephone and mail inquiries. Requests for assistance with planning for the widespread adoption of the birth center concept have come from state health department personnel and the federal government. In response we have elaborated what are to us the critical principles for establishment and operation of a birth center.[17]

Summary

The development of the Childbearing Center has been a long, difficult labor. But like childbirth it has had some moments of extreme joy. The birth of Ian, our first in-house baby, was one of those. The satisfaction of parents and staff in being able to realize each other's ideals brings continuing pleasure. The CbC was developed as a model; it is proving itself capable of meeting its stated goals of providing safe, satisfying, and economic care to carefully screened families who are anticipating a normal childbearing experience. It is also demonstrating that a system which includes those served in decision making and which is based on midwifery management of carefully screened, healthy families, backed by skilled obstetric management in the event of complications, offers our nation the most effective route to providing prevention-oriented excellence in maternity care.

CONCLUSION

Although the programs briefly described in this chapter are representative of some approaches to childbirth in the United States, there is no intention of implying that they are either the first or the best. In each region of the country innovative programs are developing. A few of the better known of these are St. Ann's Hospital, Columbus, Ohio; Booth Memorial, Philadelphia and Cleveland; Family Hospital, Milwaukee; Roosevelt Hospital, New York; St. Joseph's Hospital, Phoenix; and San Francisco General Hospital.

REFERENCES

1. Arms, S.: Immaculate deception: a new look at women and childbirth in America, Boston, 1975, Houghton Mifflin Co.
2. The Boston Women's Health Book Collective: Our bodies, ourselves: a book by and for women, New York, 1973, Simon & Schuster, Inc.
3. The case for childbirth at home, Boston Globe, Feb. 17, 1974.
4. Childbirth revolution, Harpers, **3156**:9-18, 1976.
5. Disbrow, M. A., editor: Meeting consumers' demands for maternity care, Proceedings of Conference for Nurses and Other Health Professionals, Seattle, Sept. 16, 1972.
6. Edwards, M. E.: Unattended home births, Am. J. Nurs. **73**(8):1332, 1973.
7. Elkins, V.: The rights of the pregnant parent: how to have an easier, healthier birth—together, Ottawa, Ontario, Canada, 1976, Two Continents Publishing Group.
8. Final Natality Statistics, Washington, D.C., 1969, National Center for Health Statistics, U.S. Department of Health, Education, and Welfare.
9. Gilgoff, A.: Childbirth at home, Newsday, Jan. 5, 1975.
10. Giving birth at home, New York Times, Nov. 9, 1971.
11. Haire, D.: The cultural warping of childbirth, 1972, Milwaukee, International Childbirth Education Association.
12. Hazell, L. D.: Study of 300 elective home births, Birth and Family J. **2**(1):11-18, 1975.
13. Hellman, L. M.: Nurse-midwifery in the United States, Obstet. Gynecol. **30**(6):883, 1967.
14. Hellman, L. M., and O'Brien, F. B., Jr.: Nurse-midwifery—an experiment in maternity care, Obstet. Gynecol. **24**:343-349, Sept., 1964.
15. I want my baby at home, Philadelphia Inquirer, April 14, 1974.
16. Issacs, G.: A universal model for health care or the dilemma of a primary health care agency in a medically oriented society, Paper presented at International Health Conference Program, sponsored by National Council for International Health.
17. Lubic, R. W., and Ernst, E. K.: The childbearing center: an alternative to conventional care, Nurs. Outlook **26**(12):754-760, 1978.
18. Maternity Center Association: The home birth controversy, Briefs **39**(9):134, 1975.

19. Midwives: they make house calls, Washington Star-News, Dec. 2, 1974.
20. Montgomery, T. A.: A case for nurse-midwives, Am. J. Obstet. Gynecol., vol. 105, issue 3.
21. New interest in home deliveries, Washington, D.C., Jan. 1973, Maternal and Child Health Information, Health Services Administration, Department of Health, Education, and Welfare.
22. Obstetrics seen unneeded at most normal deliveries, Ob/Gyn News 9(3):20, 1974.
23. Read, G. D.: Childbirth without fear: the principles and practice of natural childbirth, ed. 2, New York, 1959, Harper & Row Publishers.
24. The Reasoner report, ABC News, Nov. 2, 1974.
25. Shaw, N. S.: Forced labor: maternity care in the United States. In Pergamon studies in critical sociology, Elmsford, N.Y., 1974, Pergamon Press, Inc.
26. Stewart, D., and Stewart, L., editors: Safe alternatives in childbirth, Chapel Hill, N. C., 1976, National Association of Parents and Professionals for Safe Alternatives in Childbirth.

Epilogue

If you are considering changing to family-centered delivery practices using the birthing room concept, we have some suggestions for you. First, decide on your goal. If your *only* goal is to offer a homelike hospital alternative to home birth, create a separate facility. Design it with the emphasis on a decor that is as homelike as possible. In such an alternative birth setting strict admission criteria will be necessary because of the limitations on emergency intervention created by the constraints of the environment.

However, if your goal is to demystify and simplify institutions' birth rituals for almost *all* families, avoid just creating separate birthing facilities with strict admission criteria.

First, establish two birthing rooms in the regular labor and delivery area. For families delivering in these rooms, provide one-to-one labor support either from monitrices, nurses, family, friends, or other persons. In this first phase of transition, use a few basic, clear-cut criteria for family eligibility to give birth in the birthing rooms. These criteria must be such that they can be easily determined, for example, multiparas at term who have participated in prenatal education. These women should be in active labor (dilated 3 cm or more) and the fetal vertex should be engaged.

When the staff feels comfortable with this phase of the transition, move to phase two. Now add prepared nulliparas to the group eligible for birthing room births. Also continue to use the criteria of active labor and engaged vertex.

As time passes, everyone involved will gain confidence about the transition to birthing rooms. Then begin expanding criteria to include unprepared women and their families (whether nulliparas or multiparas). The goal should be individualization of criteria. Eventually, almost all families may give birth in birthing rooms, with alternative birth centers also available for the select population that meets the risk criteria.

Remember that the Manchester experience is still evolving, and allow a transition period in your implementation of alternative concepts of childbirth. Demystifying birth will be an evolutionary process in which birthing rooms replacing traditional delivery rooms for most families can play an important role.

Perhaps Don Quixote said it best*:

> Oh my friends, I have lived almost 50 years, and I have seen life as it is: pain, misery, hunger, cruelty beyond belief. I have heard the singing from taverns and the moans from bundles of filth in the street. I've been a soldier and I've seen my comrades fall in battle or die more slowly under the lash. . . . I've held them in my arms at the final moment. No glory. No gallant last words. Only their eyes filled with confusion. Whimpering the question: "Why?" I don't think they asked why they were dying, but why they had lived . . . too much sanity may be madness. *And maddest of all is to see life as it is and not as it ought to be.*

*Wasserman, D.: Man of La Mancha. In Guernsey, O. L., Jr.: The best plays of 1965-66, New York, 1966, Dodd, Mead & Co.

Joint Statement on Maternity Care (1971) and Supplementary Statement (1975)

JOINT STATEMENT ON MATERNITY CARE (1971)

The American College of Obstetricians and Gynecologists, The Nurses Association of The American College of Obstetricians and Gynecologists and the American College of Nurse-Midwives recognize the increasing needs for general health care and, more specifically, the deficits in availability and quality of maternity care. The latter, which are not confined to any social class, can best be corrected by the cooperative efforts of teams of physicians, nurse-midwives, obstetric registered nurses, and other health personnel. The composition of such teams will vary and be determined by local needs and circumstances. The functions and responsibilities of team members should be clearly defined according to the education and training of the individuals concerned.

To achieve the aims of providing optimal maternity care for all women the following recommendations are made:

1. The health team organized to provide maternity care will be directed by a qualified obstetrician-gynecologist.
2. In such medically-directed teams, qualified nurse-midwives may assume responsibility for the complete care and management of uncomplicated maternity patients.
3. In such medically-directed teams, obstetric registered nurses may assume responsibility for patient care and management according to their education, training, and experience.
4. In such medically-directed teams, other health personnel who have been trained in specific areas of maternity care may participate in the team functions according to their abilities and within the definitions of responsibility established by the team.
5. Written policies describing the specific functions of each of the team members should be prepared. They should be reviewed and revised periodically according to changing needs.

In endorsing the above statement, The American College of Obstetricians and Gynecologists, The Nurses Association of The American College of Obstetricians and Gynecologists and the American College of Nurse-Midwives recognize as their common goal the need for improvement and expansion of health services now being provided for women.

In order to maintain a continuing evaluation of the health services being provided for women and to plan for needed improvements and expansion, a mechanism for continued communication between all the organizations responsible for their provision is being developed.

SUPPLEMENTARY STATEMENT (1975)

Many questions have arisen concerning the meaning of the recommendation in the Joint Statement on Maternity Care (1971) that the health care team be "directed by a qualified obstetrician-gynecologist." These questions are justified and are accentuated by other developments in the specialty of obstetrics-gynecology, which include the changing birth rate, formalization of new roles for personnel, emphasis on preventive care, HMOs, plans for national health insurance, PSRO, and regionalization of health services.

It is recognized that the obstetrician-gynecologist cannot under all circumstances be physically present to direct the health team; therefore it is essential that mechanisms of communication be clearly established for him or her to provide direction. Thus, the nature of the direction of the health team indeed becomes crucial.

The obstetrician-gynecologist working within a team giving health care to women has many responsibilities. These range from the direct provision of services to community health efforts and include:

a. The supervision of the medical care provided by all team members
b. The direct provision of care for complications of pregnancy and for complex medical and surgical gynecological conditions
c. The setting of medical care standards
d. The provision of consultation to other team members
e. The surveillance of task distribution within the team
f. Participation in the ongoing educational activities of the team
g. The introduction of new medical techniques as they become available
h. The development of medical research*

In view of the diversity of health care systems in which the obstetric-gynecologic health team currently functions, no universal systems model can be applied. Generally, however, the team is found in the following broad contexts:

1. Urban (intramural, on site, immediate referrals)
2. Rural (with institutional affiliation)

---

*Interorganizational Committee on Ob/Gyn Health Personnel: Medical practice in the obstetric-gynecologic health care team, Sept. 1973.

3. Rural (without institutional affiliation but with obstetric consultation available)
4. Private office (urban or rural)

The logistics of consultation and referral may vary with geographic and climatic conditions, but the following basic principles of team interaction are valid regardless of these conditions:

1. There must be a written agreement among members of the team clearly specifying consultation and referral policies and standing orders. The representatives of each practice discipline should participate in the development of and be signatory to the agreement.

2. The obstetrician-gynecologist, upon signing protocols, must accept full responsibility for direction of medical care tendered by the team in accordance with his or her orders.

3. In circumstances wherein the functions of the team leader are necessarily performed by physicians without specialty training in obstetrics-gynecology, medical direction should be provided through a formal consultative arrangement with a qualified obstetrician-gynecologist who is available to team members for continuing consultation and ensurance of quality care.

Manchester monitrice class outline

A. Class I
  1. Participants' explanation of
      a. Pregnancy
      b. Labor
      c. Delivery
      d. Mental picture of themselves in labor
  2. Name of method
      a. Lamaze method of childbirth
      b. Psychoprophylactic method of childbirth
      c. Prepared childbirth
  3. Purpose of method
      a. To be aware, awake, and participatory
      b. An intelligent woman's response to a difficult task
  4. Technique achieves purpose through conditioned reflexes
  5. History of method: began in Soviet Union, to France with Dr. Lamaze, to New York and ASPO
  6. Explanation of "no failures" with the method
      a. All information learned will be of benefit
      b. No martyrs
  7. Discipline in labor
      a. Labor is hard work
      b. Need to learn discipline to learn control
  8. Pain in labor
      a. Explanation of fear-tension-pain concept
      b. Brain's ability to concentrate only on strongest stimuli
  9. Tools of method
      a. Understanding
      b. Education
      c. Exercises
      d. Breathing techniques

  e. Control of body (i.e., muscles)

 10. Talk with father

  a. He is the mother's coach and trainer

  b. Pregnancy is part of both, so the father is needed now more than ever as a helpmate

  c. Note-taking his job

 11. Introduce concept of correct posture

 12. Introduce neuromuscular exercises, beginning with father on the floor

 13. Go through *Birth Atlas*

 14. Encourage additional questions

B. Class II

 1. Review important facts of Class I, including the previously given exercises

 2. Introduce following exercises

  a. Tailor sitting

  b. String of beads

  c. Pelvic rock—fathers try this

  d. Neck and shoulder rotation

  e. Kegal's exercises

 3. General explanation of three stages of labor

 4. Introduce the very light pant; when to do slow, rhythmic chest breathing (i.e., effacement)

 5. Show slides of anatomy, leaving out the delivery until later class

C. Class III

 1. Review Class II with exercises and breathing techniques

 2. Go through three stages of labor, drawing diagrams

 3. Show breathing technique for first and second part of first stage of labor

  a. Easy breathing, slow chest

  b. Slow panting

  c. Three types of breathing

   (1) Deep slow chest—6 to 9 minutes

   (2) Rapid shallow—4/4 time (Yankee Doodle)

   (3) Pant blow—transition

 4. Introduce effleurage

 5. Explain contents and purpose of contents of paper bag

  a. Chapstick   d. Talcum powder or cornstarch

  b. Handi-Wipes e. Lollipops—sour

  c. Sponge   f. Sandwich for the father

 6. Discuss hyperventilation

D. Class IV
    1. Review exercises and breathing techniques
    2. Introduce transitional stage and the breathing technique used
    3. Explain helpful positions if back labor is present
       a. Knee-chest, squatting, kneeling, pelvic-rock
       b. Side lying with pillow under top knee
       c. Dangling with arms crossed on bedside stand top or any tabletop
       d. Father massaging sacral area, counterpressure
    4. Mention breastfeeding
       a. La Leche League
       b. Decision of mother *and* father
       c. Advantages

E. Class V
    1. Review previous class
    2. Explanation of expulsion phase
    3. Description of breathing and positioning for this phase
    4. Difference between true and false labor
    5. Show Lamaze room slides, fetal monitor

F. Class VI
    1. Review all exercises and breathing techniques
    2. Review important facts of Lamaze method
       a. Aim is to be awake, aware, and participatory
       b. Don't try to be a martyr; if medication and anesthesia needed, take without hesitation, without guilt feelings
       c. Doctor is patient's insurance and head of the team
    3. Discuss signs of impending labor
       a. Increased mucous secretions
       b. Rupture of membranes
       c. Bloody show
    4. Tell what to pack in suitcase
    5. Tell what newborn will look like
       a. Wet, wrinkled; white cheesy covering present
       b. Color
       c. Cord
       d. Explain about silver nitrate drops
    6. Touch on getting acquainted with the baby while still in the hospital and people to ask questions of; explain rooming-in
    7. Discuss circumcision
    8. Welcome any couples back for refresher class closer to their due date

Guidelines for family-centered maternity programs

OUTLINE OF THE FAMILY MATERNITY CENTER PROGRAM, MANCHESTER MEMORIAL HOSPITAL*

A. Features
1. Prenatal care by both obstetricians and nurse practitioners
2. Nutritional consultation
3. Hospital tour
4. Lecture series on pregnancy, birth, and parenting
5. Prepared childbirth classes
   a. Home classes provide warm, friendly, informal atmosphere
   b. Held weekly during last 6 weeks of pregnancy
   c. Small size (four to six couples) ensures personalized attention
   d. Certified childbirth educators
   e. Anatomy, physiology of pregnancy stressed, but all aspects of family life and relationships covered
   f. Relaxation, breathing, concentration, and proper pushing techniques taught
   g. Father (or "supporting other") actively involved
B. Recommended policies of the Family Maternity Center program
1. Family waiting room and early labor lounge, attractively painted and furnished, will be available in or near the obstetric suite where
   a. Patients in early labor can walk and visit with children, husbands, and others
   b. The support person can go for a rest break if necessary
   c. A small kitchen will be available for preparation of nourishment and snacks for the support person

---

*As approved by the Department of Obstetrics-Gynecology, Manchester Memorial Hospital, Sept. 10, 1979. Parts of the program are to be implemented when the new facilities are completed. They are currently under construction and due to be completed in 1983.

    d. Reading materials are available

    e. Telephone-intercom connections with the labor area will be available

2. A diagnostic-admitting room will be adjacent to or near the family waiting room where

    a. Women can be examined to ascertain their status in labor without being formally admitted, if they are in early labor

    b. Any woman patient past 20 weeks' gestation can be evaluated for emergency health problems during pregnancy

3. Birthing rooms

    a. Combination labor and delivery rooms for mothers and support persons during a normal labor and delivery

    b. Brightly and attractively decorated and furnished rooms designed with a homelike atmosphere; comfortable lounge chairs useful

    c. Stocked for medical emergencies for mother and infant, with equipment concealed behind wall cabinets or drapes but readily available when needed; medical technology (fetal monitors, etc.) available and used when indicated

    d. Wired for music and intercom

    e. Equipped with modern labor-delivery beds, which can be

        (1) Raised and lowered

        (2) Adjusted to semi-sitting position

        (3) Adjusted to use optional stirrups

    f. Equipped with a warmer and the capacity for infant resuscitation

    g. Appropriately supplied for normal vaginal delivery and the immediate care of newborn

    h. An environment in which breastfeeding, handling of the baby, and bonding are encouraged immediately after delivery, with due consideration given to maintaining the baby's normal temperature

4. Other labor rooms where

    a. Support persons can be with a laboring patient, whether labor is normal or abnormal, and mother is transferred to a delivery room for delivery

    b. Attention is given to the surroundings, which are attractively furnished and contain a comfortable lounge chair

5. Delivery rooms (for those not using birthing rooms)

    a. Are properly equipped with standard items

    b. Will have delivery tables with adjustable backrests to allow woman to deliver with back elevated

    c. Have an overhead mirror available

    d. Accommodate breastfeeding and handling of the baby after delivery, with due consideration given to maintaining the baby's normal temperature

6. An operating room will be available where an emergency cesarean delivery can be performed without delay
7. Recovery room (for those not using birthing room): Families may return from the delivery room or operating room to their original labor rooms, depending on the demand, or to a recovery room; such a recovery room
   a. Has all the standard equipment
   b. Allows infant to be with the mother and support persons for a time after delivery, with due consideration given to the infant's physiologic adjustment to extrauterine life
   c. Is available to postcesarean birth families, when feasible
8. The postpartum "new family unit" of the maternity center
   a. Contains flexible rooming-in with a central nursery to allow
      (1) Optional rooming-in
      (2) Babies to be returned to the central nursery for professional nursing care when desired by mother or when visitors other than immediate family are present
      (3) Maximum desired parent-infant contact, especially during the first 24 hours
   b. Has extended visiting hours for the father or "supporting other" to provide the opportunity to assist with the care and feeding of the baby
   c. Has limited visiting hours for friends, since the emphasis of the family-centered approach is on the family
   d. Contains a family (sibling visiting) room
      (1) Children can visit their mothers, fathers, and newborns
      (2) Professional staff are available to answer questions about parenting and issues regarding adjustments to the enlarged family
      (3) Cafeteria-like meals are served to mother and father
   e. Has group and individual instruction provided by appropriately prepared personnel on postpartum care, family planning, infant feeding, infant care, and parenting
   f. Encourages visiting and feeding by the mothers in special nurseries, such as
      (1) Newborn, intensive care nursery
      (2) Isolation nursery
   g. Encourages breastfeeding/bottle feeding on demand with professional personnel available for assistance
9. Discharge planning includes
   a. Options for early discharge
   b. Careful attention to continuing medical and/or nursing contact after discharge to ensure postpartum and newborn health
   c. Potential for use of appropriate referral systems

C. The advantages of the labor-delivery bed
   1. To the mother
      a. Simplicity; no physical or emotional disruptions, distractions, or dislocations
      b. Continuity of concentration and control
      c. Continuity of father and nursing support
      d. Emotionally satisfying, dignified experience
   2. To the physician (advantages for the woman are also advantages to the physician)
      a. Simplifies, expedites management
      b. Continuous supervision of vital signs, fetal monitoring, IV solutions and medication, and progress until delivery is completed
      c. Eliminates unsterile precipitous deliveries on stretcher or in delivery room
      d. Individualizes childbirth management
   3. For the nursing staff
      a. Simplifies, expedites childbirth management
      b. Eliminates the often difficult decision of when to transfer
      c. Eliminates the physical and emotional stress and strain of transfer
      d. Enables nurse to provide maximum supportive care
      e. Efficient, economic use of nursing services (no second room setup)
   4. For the administration
      a. Economy of space, staff, and time
      b. Eliminates reduplication of supplies, equipment (including fetal monitor)
      c. Less laundry and maintenance
D. Staffing pattern
   1. Regular hospital staff retained
      a. Nursing rotation between all units encouraged; labor and delivery personnel may assist personnel in postpartum and nursery areas if not needed in labor and delivery, and vice versa
      b. A minimum of one RN present in nursery at all times; additional nursery personnel assigned as needed
   2. Monitrice
      a. Supplements regular staff, thus helping to resolve the constant dilemma of "feast or famine" maternity staffing
      b. Maternity RN trained specifically in prepared childbirth techniques
      c. Provides continuous emotional and physical one-to-one support throughout labor and delivery (not necessarily available from staff nurses); reinforces but does not usurp father's role

      d. Can also be childbirth educator (combines theory with practice)

      e. 24-hour-a-day call roster

      f. Coordinates at delivery with floor nurses

      g. Not an employee of hospital; bills the parents directly

   3. "Supporting other"

      a. Could be family member in addition to father

      b. Could take place of monitrice as support person, if none available

      c. Could not assume nursing management responsibilities

E. Birth room procedures

   1. In situ delivery

   2. Birth position optional

   3. No routine episiotomy, IVs, electronic fetal monitors

   4. Mother encouraged to assist with delivery

   5. First hour post partum, parent-infant bonding encouraged

   6. Room lights dimmed post partum

   7. Silver nitrate withheld for 1 to 2 hours after birth

F. Infection control

   1. Birth rooms' bed and floor thoroughly cleaned after each birth

   2. Walls and draperies in birthing rooms cleaned once a week

   3. If mother or baby develops an infection, they are cared for according to recommendations of ACOG and state licensing agency

   4. Staff in all areas of maternity wear hospital scrub clothing while in the department (clothing is changed promptly if soiled)

   5. Strict handwashing technique is observed by all staff at all times

CONVERTING A PRIVATE LABOR ROOM TO A HOMELIKE LABOR-DELIVERY BIRTHING ROOM

The following is an outline of basic steps to follow in converting any private labor room into a homelike labor-delivery birthing room. The basic philosophy is that all "awake and aware" patients should be able to labor-deliver and have at least 1 hour post partum in the same room, assuming normal labor, thus providing individualized care in a joyous, anxiety-reducing environment.

A. Choosing and decorating room

   1. Choosing room

      a. Any room with a minimum dimension of 8 feet by 12 feet will suffice, although a slightly larger room is preferable

      b. The room may be located on obstetric floor or elsewhere in hospital, provided access to regular delivery and operating rooms is readily available

    2. Floor
      a. Any regular floor surface (tile or carpet) will suffice
      b. Conductive flooring is not necessary, since general anesthesia is not available
    3. Walls
      a. Any wall surface is acceptable; however, waterproof vinyl wallpaper is preferable because it facilitates cleaning and comes in many attractive colors (avoid white if possible)
      b. Walls should be able to accommodate hangers so that pictures, posters, bulletin boards, and other attractive features may be added.
      c. The wall at the foot of the labor-delivery bed should be able to accommodate:
        (1) A large framed mirror near the top so both mother and father can easily observe delivery
        (2) A wall-mounted Castle lamp or directional beam for visualization of perineum by obstetrician or nurse-midwife without excessive glare
      d. A wall-mounted telephone near the patient's labor-delivery bed is convenient
    4. Windows need no special treatment but should have attractive draperies on either side or curtains of the decorator's choice
    5. Ceiling
      a. May be either plaster or acoustic tile
      b. May be any color—usually white and often containing several concentration spots of various colors and design
      c. Overhead lights should use incandescent (not fluorescent) bulbs to permit postpartum dimming
B. Contents of the room
    1. Most important is a functional, versatile labor-delivery bed; we have had many years of experience with the labor-delivery bed that has been used in Europe for 2 generations, which we have found very satisfactory; advantages are that the bed
      a. Requires minimum maintenance
      b. Telescopes to one half size for delivery, thus doubling space for instrument table, etc.
      c. Has a hydraulic pump for smooth elevating and lowering of the surface of the bed by the obstetrician
      d. Has an eight-socket adjustable backrest for positioning the patient's back at various heights from the supine to the sitting position
      e. Has 30-degree Trendelenburg position readily available when necessary
      f. Has 4-inch foam cushions for comfort and patient support

g. Has two cushions in the lower section, enabling the operator to remove one or both cushions for delivery

    (1) If one cushion is removed, the foot section is pushed in halfway, permitting the mother to deliver in the semireclining position with legs at 45-degree angles and out of stirrups; or the legs may be freely placed into stirrups or out of stirrups using the single cushion as a tray for instruments following delivery of the baby during episiotomy repair

    (2) If both cushions are removed, the mother must then place her legs in the stirrups, which may be adjusted three-dimensionally by a series of elevating and lowering clamps and ball-and-socket joints

h. Has stirrups made of a comfortable, soft padded leather that support the calf and do not pinch at the knee joint; no adjustable foot support is necessary

i. May have the height individually adjusted to the desire of the operator

2. A comfortable, padded chair for the father is placed beside the head of the bed

3. The usual delivery room stool is used for the physician at the time of delivery, and the sterile instrument table and splash basin are wheeled into the room; customary sterile techniques are followed (with no increase in infection rate in 10 years experiences and over 4000 patients)

4. A Kreiselman incubator is placed in the room

5. An infant heat panel is placed parallel to the delivery table at the time of delivery and positioned over the mother's abdomen so that the parents may have sustained and continuous skin-to-skin contact with the baby without fear of hypothermia of the infant

6. An attractive wood-paneled cabinet on the wall provides a location for all appropriate medications, instruments, and other equipment for a labor-delivery room

7. Fetal monitor is used when indicated, not routinely (fetal monitrice, one-to-one continuous nursing support, *is* used routinely)

8. A private toilet is adjacent to this room; this is not a necessity but is very helpful

9. Amenities include AM-FM radio, instant camera, refrigerator for nourishment

10. Wall suction, portable oxygen

11. Birthing room log to record deliveries with comments

12. Paracervical block trays very helpful for maintaining patient comfort when necessary (mepivacaine 1% [Carbocaine])

SIBLING VISITING POLICY, MANCHESTER MEMORIAL HOSPITAL

The sibling visiting room at Manchester Memorial Hospital is intended to enhance the family experience. It is hoped that by providing such a visiting room we will help your other children accept the new baby more readily. It will reassure your other children, or child, that mother has not deserted them for the new baby. Please note the following:

1. The term "sibling" refers to your other children, not your younger brothers or sisters.
2. Only the father, a member of the immediate family, or significant "other" may accompany the siblings for visiting.
3. Siblings who visit must be screened by the maternity staff for the presence of obvious infection and permitted to visit only if found to the infection free.
4. Siblings must visit in the visiting room, not mother's room.
5. Newborn infants will be brought to the sibling visiting room where the new family can get acquainted.
6. Visiting hours are by advance appointment only and shall be scheduled for $\frac{1}{2}$ hour. On the day of sibling visiting the visit may be extended to 1 hour, provided the time period following yours has not been assigned. The nurse at the maternity desk will schedule your appointment.
7. Hours available for visiting will be:
   2 P.M. to 2:30 P.M.
   2:30 P.M. to 3 P.M.
   3 P.M. to 3:30 P.M.
   3:30 P.M. to 4 P.M.
   6:30 P.M. to 7 P.M.
   7 P.M. to 7:30 P.M.
8. Mothers who remain for an extended period may request a second sibling visit.
9. General visitors are excluded from the sibling visiting room.
10. General visiting hours
    Fathers—Anytime
    Mother's rest time—*No Visitors Allowed: 2 to 3 P.M.
    General visiting—3 P.M. to 4 P.M., 6:30 P.M. to 7:30 P.M.
    Except for siblings, children under 16 are not allowed

MANCHESTER MEMORIAL HOSPITAL
Manchester, Connecticut

POSTPARTUM OBSERVATION SHEET

STANDARD PROCEDURE:
1. Constant observation for 1 hour;
2. First hour after delivery of placenta: Observe and chart q 5 minutes pulse, fundus, bleeding; q 15 minutes B.P.
3. Second hour: Observe and chart q 15 minutes pulse, fundus, bleeding, B.P.
4. Third hour: Observe and chart q 30 minutes pulse, fundus, bleeding, B.P.

Delivery date: _____ Time: _____ at _____ M. Placenta delivered at: _____ M.

Oxytocic: _____ M. Anesthetic: _____

Time	Pulse	Fundus			Bleeding				B.P.	Medication & remarks
		Firm		Level	None	Sl.	Mod.	Prof.		
		Yes	No	(U + or −)						

LAMAZE LOG
By Manchester Monitrice Associates

Month/year	Date	Name	Doctor	Monitrice	Age	Gravida	Para	A.R.M.	IV fluids	IV oxytocin (Pitocin)	E.F.M.-Ext.	E.F.M.-Int.	Induction	Medication	Anesthesia

*F = Father in OR; type of delivery: SP = spontaneous, VE = vacuum extractor, LF = low
CS, give reason; describe complications if any.

Type of delivery	Episiotomy	Birthing room	Trans. to del. room	OR-CS (H)	Hrs. in hospital	Time of delivery	Weight	Sex	30 min. temp.	Baby Apgar mins. 1	5	Comments*	Monitrice hrs.

forceps; anesthesia: Pc = paracervical block, Pd = pudenal block; if induction, give reason; if

APPENDIX D

Early pregnancy class series

There are three sessions, each 2½ hours long.

SESSION ONE

GOALS

1. To present basic information on the female reproductive system, menstrual cycle, and conception
2. To explain normal body changes during early pregnancy and comfort measures to cope with these changes
3. To encourge discussion of emotional changes during pregnancy

OBJECTIVES: at the end of this session the participants will be able to:

1. Identify the uterus, fallopian tubes, ovaries, vagina, bladder, uterine ligaments, and rectum when shown diagrams of these anatomic parts
2. Explain one function of each of the following: uterus, ovaries, fallopian tubes, vagina
3. Identify the uterine fundus and cervix when shown a diagram
4. Point out the fertile period when given a calendar of a normal menstrual cycle
5. Define fertilization
6. Identify the part of the uterus where the fertilized ovum usually implants
7. Calculate their own estimated date of conception (EDC) according to Nagele's rule
8. List three reasons for prenatal exams
9. List one change due to pregnancy for each of the following body systems: genitourinary (GU) and gastrointestinal (GI)
10. Suggest at least one way to cope with minor changes in the GU and GI systems during early pregnancy
11. Explain how attitudes toward the pregnancy may change as the pregnancy progresses
12. Discuss male and female sexuality during pregnancy
13. Discuss role changes that occur in becoming parents
14. Demonstrate body mechanics and comfort measures for use during early pregnancy

196

Pregnancy as a normal function

A. Reproductive system
 1. Anatomic vocabulary of pregnancy
 2. Functions
B. Menstrual cycle
 1. Hormones
 2. Fertile period
C. Conception
 1. Fertilization
 2. Implantation
D. EDC
 1. Calculation
 2. Normal range
E. Prenatal examinations
 1. Importance
 2. Explanation of procedures

Normal body changes

A. Body systems
 1. GU: urinary frequency
 2. GI
    a. Nausea and vomiting
    b. Heartburn
 3. Reproductive
    a. Braxton Hicks' contractions
    b. Breast fullness
    c. Uterine size
    d. Vaginal discharge
B. Coping with minor discomforts
 1. Personal hygiene
 2. Clothing
 3. Breast care and supportive bra
 4. Vaginal discharge
 5. Recreation and travel

Emotional changes during pregnancy

A. Changes in body image
 1. Female
 2. Male
B. Attitudes (from ambivalence to acceptance)

   C. Sexuality
       1. Needs changes
           a. Female
           b. Male
       2. Myths and taboos: intercourse
   D. Role changes
       1. Mothering
       2. Fathering
       3. Parenting

Exercises: comfort techniques and body mechanics for pregnancy demonstrated

SESSION TWO

GOALS
   1. To present basic information on the composition and function of the placenta
   2. To provide information on fetal growth and status
   3. To promote awareness of danger signs of pregnancy
   4. To increase awareness of dangers of self-medication, smoking, and substance abuse during pregnancy
   5. To increase awareness of effect of pregnancy on the family constellation (grandparents, siblings, etc.)
OBJECTIVES: by the end of this session the participants will be able to:
   1. List three functions of the placenta
   2. Identify the normal range of fetal heart tone (FHT)
   3. Define presentation and position
   4. Identify the height of the uterine fundus at 20 weeks', 38 weeks', and 40 weeks' gestation
   5. Discuss the probability of fetal survival outside of the uterus at 28 weeks', 32 weeks', 36 weeks', and 40 weeks' gestation
   6. Explain the effect of maternal smoking during pregnancy on the growing fetus
   7. Discuss the effect of alcohol intake during pregnancy on the growing fetus
   8. Identify "acceptable" amounts of alcohol intake during pregnancy
   9. Discuss changing total-family roles and responsibilities

Fetal growth and status

   A. Presentation and position
   B. FHT
   C. Height of fundus
   D. Fetal development

  E. Fetus as a person
    1. Sucking
    2. Drinking
    3. Urinating
    4. Movement

Self-medication

  A. Smoking
  B. Over-the-counter drugs: aspirin
  C. Prescription drugs
  D. Alcohol
  E. Street drugs
  F. X-ray examinations: dental, chest examination, etc.

Danger signs

  A. Spotting, bleeding
  B. Cramping, pain
  C. Preeclampsia
  D. Headache, excessive swelling, blurred vision

Family

  A. Grandparents; roles
  B. Siblings
    1. Rivalry
    2. Acceptance
  C. Other members

SESSION THREE

GOALS
  1. To promote knowledge of basic dietetic habits for pregnancy and lactation
  2. To encourage practice of sound nutritional habits for each participant
  3. To present information concerning methods of feeding baby
  4. To increase awareness of resources available for families in the childbearing cycle

OBJECTIVES: at the end of this session, the participants will be able to:
  1. Identify normal weight gain during pregnancy
  2. Define "good nutrition"
  3. List four basic food groups
  4. Describe their own average daily diet in terms of grams of protein content

    5. Identify four foods high in complete proteins
    6. List four foods high in iron content
    7. Differentiate between complete and incomplete proteins
    8. List two pros and two cons for both breast and bottle feeding
    9. Discuss preparation of the breasts for breastfeeding
  10. Discuss preparations necessary for bottle feeding
  11. List at least two community resources for pregnancy support
  12. Demonstrate exercises for relaxation and pelvic floor support

Good nutrition as a family concern

    A. Importance in life cycle
    B. Value in pregnancy and lactation
    C. Weight gain

Food elements stressed in pregnancy and lactation

    A. Pregnancy diet
    B. Diet histories and inventories
    C. Food composition and quality

Supplements and restrictions

    A. Prenatal capsules
    B. Fluids
    C. Special diets
       1. Lactose intolerance
       2. Vegetarian
       3. Ethnic foods

Emotions and eating (psychology of eating)

Methods of feeding baby

    A. Breast
       1. Pros and cons
       2. Preparation
    B. Bottle
       1. Pros and cons
       2. Preparation

Resources available

A. Educational
B. Dental
C. Medical
D. Social
E. Emergency
F. Community

Exercises: relaxation techniques and Kegal's (pelvic floor) exercises demonstrated

Refresher course in childbirth preparation

There are three sessions, each 2¹/₂ hours long.

GOALS
1. To provide the participants with a review of the birth process and exercises that will aid them in labor and delivery
2. To encourage discussion of changing family roles and family adjustments

OBJECTIVES
1. To facilitate discussion of participants' previous birth experiences in an attempt to resolve unanswered questions
2. To provide a review of normal pregnancy, labor, delivery, and immediate postpartum period
3. To promote awareness of the team concept for labor
4. To provide information on alternatives available for labor and delivery
5. To provide a review of variations from normal labor
6. To provide a review of relaxation techniques, breathing techniques, and other coping techniques for labor and delivery
7. To encourage discussion of parent-infant attachment
8. To promote awareness of changing personal needs as family grows

SESSION ONE

A. Introduction to teacher and each other
   1. Teacher introduction
   2. Participants' introduction
      a. Present pregnancy
      b. Past pregnancy, labor, and birth
   3. Presentation of course outline
   4. Discussion
      a. Questions
      b. Answers
B. Pregnancy review
   1. Common terminology
   2. Fertilization

   3. Implantation
   4. EDC
   5. Body changes
C. Multipara labor
   1. Stages of labor
   2. Normal labor pattern
   3. Variations from normal labor
D. Coping techniques for labor
   1. Normal labor
   2. Back labor
   3. Induced or augmented labor

SESSION TWO

A. Review of previous class
   1. Questions
   2. Answers
   3. Discussion
B. Alternatives available for labor and delivery
   1. Team support
   2. Ambulation
   3. Analgesia
   4. Anesthesia
   5. Environmental concerns
      a. Lights
      b. Noise
      c. Positions
      d. Photographs
C. Multipara delivery
   1. Normal
   2. Variations
   3. Cesarean birth
D. Coping techniques for delivery
   1. Pushing
   2. Perineal relaxation and release

SESSION THREE

A. Review of previous class
   1. Questions
   2. Answers
   3. Discussion

B. Parent-infant attachment
   1. Defined
   2. Implications
   3. Importance
C. Review of postpartum period
   1. Normal physiology
   2. Variations
D. Family adjustments
   1. Siblings
   2. Parents
   3. Roles
E. Practice all breathing techniques for labor and delivery
   1. Review
   2. Summary

Index

A

Admission procedures for alternative birth center, 143-147

Africa, east, birth environment in, 3

After-birth celebration, 33-34, 40

Allgemeines Krankenhaus (Vienna), 6-7

Alternative birth center; see Birth center, alternative

Alternative maternity care, defined, 168

Ambulation in labor, 64

American Board of Obstetrics and Gynecology, 9

American College of Nurse-Midwives, 179

American College of Obstetricians and Gynecologists, 179

American Hospital Association, *Patient's Bill of Rights*, 97

American Indian cultures, birth in, 2, 3

American Society for Psychoprophylaxis in Obstetrics, 13, 120

Anesthesia
  and medication, 30
  paracervical block, 130-133
  used for multiparas in birthing room, 43, 44
  used for nulliparas in birthing room, 43, 44

Apparel of staff in birthing rooms, 135

Astor, Mrs. John Jacob, 8

Attachment, 60-61

Attitudes and behavior
  change of, theories of, 102
  relation of, 101

B

Barbiturates, 65

Behavior
  and attitudes
    changes of, theories of, 102
    relation of, 101
  human, relation of to change, 100-102

Beliefs, 101

Belvedere Hospital (Paris), 13-14

Bing, Elisabeth, 120

Birth
  couple active in, 16, 17
  historical role of men and fathers in, 2-3

Birth—cont'd
  length of stay in hospital after, 133-134
  positions and furniture during, 4-5
  preparation for, refresher course in, 202-204
  in primitive societies, 1-2
    abnormal, 3-4
  sibling visitation after, 136
  in underdeveloped areas, 10

Birth center
  alternative, 139-175
    admission procedures for, 143-147
    certified nurse-midwives at, 148, 150
    and discharge orders for home care, 144
    early discharge from, for newborn, 144
    high-risk factors developing after admission to, 141-142
    high-risk factors excluding admission to, 139-141
    and home visits, 144-146
    nursing procedures for, 143-147
    at Santa Cruz (California) Community Hospital, 160, 166
  family
    achievement of goals in, 157-158
    appropriate room for, 151-153
    delivery in, 156
    early discharge from, 156-157
    labor in, 155-156
    at Los Gatos (California) Community Hospital, 151-158
    medical barriers to, 151
    nonmedical barriers to, 150-151
    preparation of parents for, 155
    staff for, 154-155
    transformation of Manchester Memorial Hospital's maternity unit into, 40-46

Birth choices, other, 139-175

Birth environment, 3-4, 72-73
  decorum in choice of, 5
  historical background of, 1-11

Birth experience
  and father attachment, 58
  of parents, 53-54

Birth memories, 48

Birth rituals, demystifying and simplifying, 177-178